*Jack E. Fincham, PhD, RPh*

# Taking Your Medicine
## *A Guide to Medication Regimens and Compliance for Patients and Caregivers*

*Pre-publication*
REVIEWS,
COMMENTARIES,
EVALUATIONS . . .

"**M**uch more than a simple guide-book for helping patients improve their medication compliance, this book presents patients and their caregivers with an approach to becoming more active partners in their health care. It is a guidebook on how to become an intelligent and effective user of medications.

Chapters are devoted not only to compliance issues (e.g., why compliance is important, tools to improve compliance, reasons for not complying), but also cover the broader issue of good medication practices. Information is provided on why drugs are prescribed, how to choose a pharmacist, informing health professionals about your health, dangerous drug interactions, how to take medications, and how to help aging parents with their medication use. A sum-mary chapter highlights and reinforces the most important ideas and points.

Throughout the text are 'key point' boxes which are very helpful and action-oriented so patients can become motivated to make changes in their compliance behavior. Also included are many useful tables on topics such as medical abbreviations, finding medication assistance programs, and quality Web sites for locating additional information.

This book is loaded with helpful ideas and strategies to achieve good medication use. It is not only useful for patients and their caregivers; it should also be read by pharmacists, other health care providers, and students in the health professions."

**Michael Montagne, PhD**
*Professor of Social Pharmacy,*
*Department of Pharmaceutical Sciences,*
*Massachusetts College of Pharmacy*

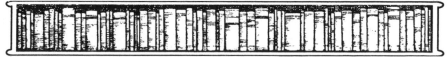

*More pre-publication*
*REVIEWS, COMMENTARIES, EVALUATIONS . . .*

"This easy-to-read book provides an insightful examination of medication compliance written for the patient/consumer from the perspective of the pharmacist. Dr. Fincham is nationally recognized in medication compliance and behavioral medicine, and is well qualified to write this important book. The book is written to help you and yours become healthier by taking medications easier and becoming more compliant with drug regimens.

The problem of medication compliance may be the most important issue affecting physicians, pharmacists, and patients today. This book is a valuable addition to bookshelves of consumers who want to learn how to use their medications in a safe and cost-effective way. Pharmacists and physicians will also be interested in this book if their goal is to reduce prescription drug costs and overall health care costs. Given the escalating cost of drugs, the need today for this book is crucial."

**David M. Scott, MPH, PhD, RPh**
*Associate Professor of Pharmacy Administration, Department of Pharmacy Practice, College of Pharmacy, North Dakota State University*

"Most of us do not enjoy the luxury of having a doctor in our homes to answer our questions about how to safely use and properly understand our prescription medicines. Now, however, we can have with us the knowledge of one of America's finest pharmacists. In this book, Dr. Fincham has provided a valuable resource to understand the sometimes cryptic world of medicine. This wonderfully written primer will help you 'take your medicine' with confidence."

**Robert R. Broadbooks, DD, MDiv**
*District Superintendent, Tennessee District Church of the Nazarene*

Pharmaceutical Products Press®
An Imprint of The Haworth Press, Inc.
New York • London • Oxford

# Taking Your Medicine
## *A Guide to Medication Regimens and Compliance for Patients and Caregivers*

# PHARMACEUTICAL PRODUCTS PRESS®
## Titles of Related Interest

*Pharmacy Ethics* edited by Mickey Smith, Steven Strauss, H. John Baldwin, and Kelly T. Alberts

*Advancing Prescription Medicine Compliance: New Paradigms, New Practices* edited by Jack E. Fincham

*A History of Nonprescription Product Regulation* by W. Steven Pray

*Pharmacy and the U.S. Health Care System, Third Edition* edited by Michael Ira Smith, Albert I. Wertheimer, and Jack E. Fincham

*Prescribed Medications and the Public Health: Laying the Foundation for Risk Reduction* by William N. Kelly

# Taking Your Medicine
## *A Guide to Medication Regimens and Compliance for Patients and Caregivers*

Jack E. Fincham, PhD, RPh

Pharmaceutical Products Press®
An Imprint of The Haworth Press, Inc.
New York • London • Oxford

For more information on this book or to order, visit
http://www.haworthpress.com/store/product.asp?sku=5579

or call 1-800-HAWORTH (800-429-6784) in the United States and Canada
or (607) 722-5857 outside the United States and Canada

or contact orders@HaworthPress.com

Published by

Pharmaceutical Products Press®, an imprint of The Haworth Press, Inc., 10 Alice Street, Binghamton, NY 13904-1580.

PUBLISHER'S NOTE
**This book has been published solely for educational purposes and is not intended to substitute for the medical advice of a treating physician.** Medicine is an ever-changing science. As new research and clinical experience broaden our knowledge, changes in treatment may be required. While many potential treatment options are made herein, some or all of the options may not be applicable to a particular individual. Therefore, the author, editor, and publisher do not accept responsibility in the event of negative consequences incurred as a result of the information presented in this book. We do not claim that this information is necessarily accurate by the rigid scientific and regulatory standards applied for medical treatment. **No warranty, expressed or implied, is furnished with respect to the material contained in this book. The reader is urged to consult with his/her personal physician with respect to the treatment of any medical condition.**

Cover design by Jennifer M. Gaska.

**Library of Congress Cataloging-in-Publication Data**

Fincham, Jack E.
    Taking your medicine : a guide to medication regimens and compliance for patients and caregivers / Jack E. Fincham.
       p. cm.
    Includes bibliographical references and index.
    ISBN-13: 978-0-7890-2858-7 (hc. : alk. paper)
    ISBN-10: 0-7890-2858-1 (hc. : alk. paper)
    ISBN-13: 978-0-7890-2859-4 (pbk. : alk. paper)
    ISBN-10: 0-7890-2859-X (pbk. : alk. paper)
    1. Chemotherapy. 2. Patient compliance. 3. Drugs—Prescribing. 4. Medical personnel and patient. I. Title.

    RM263.F55 2005
    615.5'8—dc22
                                                                                   2005007982

To Melinda, Kelcie, Derek, and Joni—
thank you for all your love, support,
and encouragement

# ABOUT THE AUTHOR

**Jack E. Fincham, PhD, RPh,** is the A.W. Jowdy Professor of Pharmacy Care at the University of Georgia College of Pharmacy in Athens, and is a member of the Nonprescription Drug Advisory Committee of the United States Food and Drug Administration. From 1994 to 2004, he served as Dean of the University of Kansas School of Pharmacy in Lawrence, and in 1998, he was named one of the top 50 most influential pharmacists in the United States by *Drug Topics* magazine. Dr. Fincham has authored more than 200 refereed and professional manuscripts, published in more than 50 journals, and has made more than 200 professional and research presentations to domestic and international groups.

# CONTENTS

# Introduction

This book will provide you with some simple ideas that can easily be implemented to help you or those you care for. You may be reading this book to help yourself be compliant, or you may wish to help a loved one (spouse, child, parent, or grandparent) better comply with prescription instructions. This book will give you tips that you can use right away to become more compliant in taking medications.

If you or someone you take care of or care for has trouble remembering to take scheduled doses of prescribed drugs, you or they are not alone. Taking drugs on a regularly scheduled basis is a difficult task. Many things occur in our lives that divert our attention to other pressing matters. In fact, 50 percent of us are noncompliant with prescription instructions at some point. It is so easy to be critical of ourselves or others that have trouble with taking medications as scheduled, but be gentle. Many times the dosing and frequency of administration of drugs can be confusing.

This book is written to help you better understand the process of taking medications and to *help you or someone you care for* learn how to be compliant with drug regimens. It is sometimes difficult to be compliant with medications because you have so many other important things to deal with on a day-to-day basis. However, medication compliance can save you time, money, and future health care problems.

Health providers are critical of patients who do not comply with regimens. The words used to describe those of us who are struggling to take medications as prescribed include

- noncompliant
- noncooperative
- deviant
- forgetful
- nonadherent

We all need to worry less about labeling patients and more about helping understand and solve the problem of medication noncompliance. I vividly recall asking a woman in her nineties about her drug-taking and compliance behavior. I wanted to find out how and when she became noncompliant with her blood pressure medication. I asked: "When did you take your medications today, and did you forget to take some of the doses?" Her reply was swift and insightful: "Listen, how can you expect me to know about something I forgot to do in the first place?" What a great answer this was—one that embarrassed me more than a little. The lesson learned was simple: rather than blaming them for not being compliant, learn to help patients learn how to help themselves become as compliant as they can be.

Anything that we do to improve compliance will rarely be 100 percent successful. However, most things that we do to become more compliant can improve our health. That is the goal of this book—how to help you and yours become healthier by making the medication taking easier and thus making it easier to be compliant with drug regimens.

Within the chapters, key points summarize important factors to consider when you take or give medications. These points can provide immediate help to you and your loved ones as you try to comply with medication schedules. An appendix at the end of the book provides specific Web site and further drug-related information for seniors, drug-related information for parents and children, and a listing of numerous Web sites containing information about drugs for all age groups.

The tips included in this book hopefully will provide you with some definite actions to take right away to improve your health. You are the most important person in the health care system, and you are the person this book is written for. Let us start today to be healthier by helping ourselves as much as we can with the drugs that we take.

# Chapter 1

# Why Drugs Are Prescribed

Drugs* have the ability to ease suffering, help control disease, and in some cases actually provide a cure for patients. Various types of drugs or medications have been ordered for patients for thousands of years. For centuries, the mainstay of drug therapies was drugs derived from plant sources. One of the most widely used drugs for the treatment of congestive heart failure is digoxin, a drug extracted from *Digitalis lanata* (foxglove). The medical use of digoxin was first advocated by Dr. William Withering,[1] who used the drug from foxglove plants in the garden of the "witch woman of Shropshire" in England. The first use was as a treatment for dropsy.

It was not until the mid-twentieth century that drugs manufactured on a large scale became commonplace and widely used. The "new age" of pharmacy was ushered in shortly after World War II when the antibiotic penicillin was mass-produced and introduced for widespread use. Later, the introduction of drugs such as chlorpromazine in the early 1960s, used to treat mental disorders (psychoses, psychotic episodes), revolutionized the treatment of the mentally ill in the United States and the world. Also in the 1960s, the entry of the drug levodopa into the marketplace revolutionized the treatment of Parkinson's disease. Drugs to treat heart ailments, cancer, diabetes, and infectious diseases are much in demand. As the demand for pharmaceuticals has risen, so have the prices and profits of the pharmaceutical industry. It is not uncommon for the percentage increase in the price of drugs to rise by double digits each year.

Prescription medications are expensive. Inflation in the cost of prescription drugs has outpaced the rate of inflation for other health care

---

*Throughout this book, the terms *drug* and *medication* will be used interchangeably. When I use the word *drug,* it is in reference to a legitimate medication used for therapeutic purposes.

goods and services in the recent past. Future price increases are also expected to be higher for pharmaceuticals than for other health care services. These facts alone require careful consideration by patients when taking medications.

Insurance coverage for prescription drugs is also spotty, and many Americans find that they have no insurance coverage for drugs. Or, it may be that the insurance that you have covers only a portion of your total drug costs.

However, being compliant with both short- and long-term medications can save future expenses for other costly drugs or medical care services. The effective use of drugs can help individuals avoid hospitalization, surgery, or other medical procedures. Through the avoidance of costly and invasive procedures, spending money for drugs can help make up for the initial outlay of funds required for their purchase. Drugs taken daily for chronic diseases, such as high blood pressure, can help patients maintain health equilibrium even though they have a chronic disease. The use of antibiotics to treat infections has allowed patients to take short courses of drug therapies and eliminate bacterial infections within weeks. Countless lives have been saved and the quality of life improved for many through the use of drugs.

## *TYPES OF DRUGS*

In the United States medications are divided into two classes: prescription and non-prescription (or over-the-counter [OTC]) drugs. Any new drug can be submitted for approval as a prescription or OTC medication; however, virtually all new drugs in the United States enter the market as a prescription drug product. After use of the drug occurs over a period of years, the manufacturing company can petition the United States Food and Drug Administration (FDA) to switch the product from prescription to OTC status.

---

### KEY POINT

*Make sure that your doctor and pharmacist know all the medications that you are taking. These may be prescription, OTC, or herbal products. Regardless of the type of medication, let your caregivers know all the drugs that you regularly take.*

---

Drugs are available to treat many chronic and acute conditions. Many older and newer drugs are available to treat conditions listed in Exhibits 1.1 and 1.2. These lists are not all-inclusive, but they do contain the more commonly seen conditions. Treating these conditions may include the use of prescription and OTC drugs.

---

### KEY POINT

*Never accept the directions "take as directed" or "as directed" on your prescriptions. Your physician and pharmacist need to explain in detail how you are to take any medicine. Keep asking until you receive proper directions.*

---

With the potential to ease suffering comes the potential to also cause side effects, adverse effects, or provide no help whatsoever. Side effects to medications are not only aggravating; they are a first indicator that something is wrong. Do not assume when an adverse effect occurs that there is something you are doing wrong or that it is your fault. You know your body better than anyone, so if something does not seem right and you are taking a medication (new or long-term), contact your physician or pharmacist. Always let one or both of them know what is happening with the drugs you take and the effects that they have on you.

**EXHIBIT 1.1. Examples of chronic diseases that are treated with drugs.**

Allergies
Alzheimer's disease
Arthritis
Asthma
Benign prostatic hypertrophy (BPH)
Blood clots
Bronchitis
Certain types of cancers
Chronic pain
Congestive heart failure (heart failure)
Depression
Emphysema
Erectile dysfunction
Gout
High blood pressure (hypertension)
High blood sugar (diabetes)
High cholesterol (hyperlipidemia)
Lung congestion
Osteoporosis
Parkinson's disease
Psychoses
Raynaud's syndrome
Vitamin deficiencies

**EXHIBIT 1.2. Examples of acute conditions treated with drugs.**

Anxiety
Athlete's foot (tinea pedis)
Certain types of cancers
Fluid retention
Gastroesophageal reflux disorder
Headaches
Hemorrhoids
Infections
- Skin (lesions, cuts, abrasions that have become infected)
- Systemic (lungs, urinary tract, kidney)
- Upper respiratory tract
- Viral (common cold)

Influenza
Insect sting
Insomnia
Nasal congestion
Seasonal allergies
Skin irritation
Skin rash
- Diaper rash (severe)

## KEY POINT

*Side effects, or adverse effects, to drug therapy are commonplace. If you experience a change in how your feel, your bodily functions, or a dramatic decline in your functioning, contact your physician or pharmacist immediately. Side effects can occur with any medication, even those you have taken for extended periods of time.*

## Nutritional Supplements Are Drugs

Remember that the herbal and nutritional supplements you take are drugs too. They may not be regulated the way prescription and OTC medications are, but they also have the potential to bring you help or harm. Know what is in the supplements that you take and be aware of their effect on how you feel and how you function. If you feel that something is just not right, it probably is not. Find out as much as you can from reliable sources about the supplements and what they can and cannot accomplish. Ask questions of your health providers. Be relentless in obtaining this information. If you cannot find someone who is knowledgeable about these nutritional supplements, seek help on your own from books, the Internet, or other health providers.

**KEY POINT**

*Herbal supplements and nutritional products are drugs. Seek information on the products you are taking, pay attention to their effects on you, and find out how they may interact with other drugs you are taking.*

## THE PRESCRIPTION AND WHAT IT MEANS

Some of the symbols on a written prescription sheet that you receive from your physician are centuries old, and some of the symbols may be fairly new, but all need to be understandable by the pharmacist who fills your prescription. See Figure 1.1 for an example of what a prescription blank may look like.

The symbol ℞ that is always somewhere on your written prescription is ancient. Several theories have been suggested about the symbol's origin. Rx is an abbreviation for the Latin word *recipere,* which means "to take" or "to take thus." Centuries ago, this would have been a direction to a pharmacist, and would precede the recipe for a drug. There is also a theory that the shape of the symbol is representative of the Eye of Horus.[2,3] Horus was the Egyptian god of the sky, light, and goodness. He was the son of Isis, the nature goddess, and Osiris, the god of the underworld. Osiris was murdered by his brother Seth, the god of darkness and evil. Horus sought to avenge the death of his father by challenging Seth to a fight. Seth cut out Horus's eye, but Thoth, a god associated with wisdom and compassion, magically restored it. Horus's eye then became a symbol for health (see Figure 1.2). In examining the symbol of the eye of Horus, you can see the elements of the symbol ℞.[4]

### What All the Writing Means

On the prescription form depicted in Figure 1.1 are several components telling the pharmacist what to do with this order. There is obviously a listing of a drug or, in the case of a compounded prescription, a listing of all ingredients that the physician wants included in the preparation. So, for the main part of the prescription you will have the following components listed:

1. The drug
2. The quantity to be dispensed
3. The directions for taking the medication (sig. or signature)

The physician signs the prescription and indicates how many times the prescription can be refilled (number of refills allowed), if any.

---

**J. J. Burke, M.D.**
**123 Street Drive**
**Someplace, GA 30306**
**(706) 555-1212**

Name ___[Your name here]___  Age _____

Address ___[Your address here]___  Date _____

# Rx

[Drug name here] **Lipitor**

[Quantity to be dispensed] **# 30**

[Directions for use] **Sig: Take one tablet daily**

Dispense As Written
Refill __XX__ Times

___[Doctor signs here]___
J. J. Burke, MD

DEA No. _____

---

FIGURE 1.1. Example of a prescription.

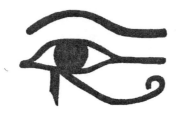

FIGURE 1.2. The eye of Horus.

Most states now mandate that there be two lines for signature on the prescription: one to indicate whether the drug can be substituted with a generic product, and the second to indicate whether only the brand-name product is to be used in filling the prescription. There may also be a DEA number—the U.S. Drug Enforcement Administration requires that physicians have a DEA number before they are allowed to write prescriptions for controlled substances in the United States. These controlled substances include potentially abused drugs such as codeine, morphine, hydrocodone, oxycodone, diazepam, alprazolam, and barbiturates, among many other substances.

Numerous abbreviations appear on a prescription. Pharmacists decipher all of these symbols and abbreviations or, if they cannot, they will not hesitate to contact the doctor to clarify the information! Table 1.1 presents some common abbreviations and directive segments that physicians use to instruct the patient on how the prescription is to be taken.

---

**KEY POINT**

*If you cannot read the written prescription that the doctor writes for you, your pharmacist may not be able to either. Make sure you ask what drugs are being prescribed for you and see if they match the condition for which you sought treatment.*

---

### Filling the Prescription

You can take your prescription to any pharmacy for filling. For certain insurance plans, you may have to use a mail-order pharmacy to have your prescriptions filled. There may be exceptions to this re-

TABLE 1.1. Some common abbreviations appearing on prescriptions and their meanings.

| Standard abbreviations | Definition/Dosing schedule* | Comments |
|---|---|---|
| QDAY, QD, Q.D. | To be taken once daily | I suggest taking at 9 a.m. |
| QAM, qam | To be taken once daily in the morning | I suggest taking at 9 a.m. |
| Daily | To be taken once daily | I suggest taking at 9 a.m. |
| QHS, q hs | To be taken once daily at bedtime | I suggest taking between 9 and 11 p.m. |
| QPM, q pm | To be taken once daily in the evening | I suggest taking at 9 p.m. |
| BID, b.i.d. | To be taken twice daily | I suggest taking at 9 a.m. and 9 p.m. |
| TID, t.i.d. | To be taken three times a day | I suggest taking at 9 a.m., 3 p.m., and 9 p.m. |
| TID AC, t.i.d. a.c. | To be taken three times a day, before meals | I suggest taking at 7 a.m., 11 a.m., and 5 p.m. This assumes that you normally eat at 8 a.m., 12 noon, and 6 p.m. If your schedule is different for meals, just plan on taking the doses one hour before you eat your regular meals. |
| TID PC, t.i.d. p.c. | To be taken three times a day with meals or with a snack (crackers, etc.) | I suggest taking at your normal meal times. |
| AC HS, a.c. h.s. | To be taken before meals and at bedtime | I suggest taking at 7 a.m., 11 a.m., 5 p.m., and 9 p.m. |
| QID, q.i.d. | To be taken four times a day | I suggest 9 a.m., 1 p.m., 5 p.m., and 9 p.m. |
| PRN, p.r.n. | To be taken as needed | I suggest caution with this dosing regimen. Please make sure that you know the maximum number of doses that you can take daily. Physicians and pharmacists assume that patients know how many doses can be taken. This is not always the case; ask them to tell you the number of doses that can be safely consumed in one day. With pain medications, it may be that you need to consume several doses throughout the day; with a medication to help you sleep, you should take just one dose. |

| | | |
|---|---|---|
| Q 6 hours, q 6 h | To be taken every six hours | I suggest taking at 6 a.m., 12 noon, 6 p.m., and 12 midnight. |
| Q 8 hours, q 8 h | To be taken every eight hours | I suggest taking at 8 a.m., 4 p.m., and 12 midnight. |
| Q 12 hours, q 12 h | To be taken every twelve hours | I suggest taking at 9 a.m. and 9 p.m. |
| a.c. | Before meals | |
| p.c. | After meals | |
| q.o.d. | Every other day | |
| o.u. | Both eyes | |
| o.d. | Right eye | |
| o.s. | Left eye | |
| a.u. | Both ears | |
| a.d. | Right ear | |
| a.s. | Left ear | |
| gtts. | Drops | |
| p.o. | By mouth, orally | |

*With any dosing instructions, your physician may specifically let you know when the dose should be taken; often, however, patients are left on their own to determine the dosing schedule for their medications.

quirement for prescriptions that must be filled immediately (e.g., for antibiotics, pain medications, muscle relaxants, etc.). Other requirements may affect you depending on the type of health insurance coverage that you have. For example, if you are eligible for U.S. Veterans Administration (VA) coverage, VA pharmacies will be used to fill your prescriptions. Other pharmacies may not accept the insurance program that you have for your drug benefit, but this is extremely rare.

You have the right to use any pharmacy and can change pharmacies at any time. You should be able to do this without any trouble; pharmacies transfer prescriptions all the time. Your pharmacist can do this for you easily. This is very handy to know if you are traveling or perhaps moving to a different part of the country.

## YOUR RIGHTS CONCERNING
## PHARMACISTS AND PHYSICIANS

You have a right to be treated fairly and courteously by your health providers. You should have access to your physicians and pharmacists when you have a question or concern. It may be difficult to reach your physician via phone, but mechanisms should be available to allow them to phone you back at a more convenient time if they are busy at the time you call. Also, office and staff nurses are a wonderful resource for questions and help. The way most medical practices are set up, it is usually more convenient to phone a nurse with questions; they can respond themselves or have the physician contact you.

Pharmacists are no doubt the most accessible of any of the health professionals in the United States. Most are easily accessible in person or by phone. Computer answering and screening machines are used everywhere (and by everyone, it seems) in the United States, but through a relatively easy process, most pharmacists can be reached quickly and should be able to speak with you should the need arise.

In my opinion, accessibility of your doctor or pharmacist is *not* an optional service. These individuals should be accessible and able to answer questions that you have. Your health is your most important attribute, and to take the best possible care of yourself, you need to be able to have questions answered. Often in physicians' offices it is easy to be distracted and forget to ask questions that you feel are important. It might help you to do the following:

1. Write down all your questions before you visit your doctor.
2. Take this written sheet to the appointment with your doctor.
3. Make a copy of the sheet and provide the nurse that first sees you with the questions.
4. Tell a loved one about your list and have him or her remind you of what you wanted to ask.
5. Write down all the drugs that you take; make sure the doctor sees this list.
6. Have someone go to the appointment with you.
7. Follow up afterward to ensure that you have remembered all the questions and have the answers that you need.
8. Ask again if you did not receive the answers that you need to understand treatments, therapies, drugs, and so on.

9. When you see a physician or pharmacist, you are the most important person in the encounter; make sure you find out what you need to know.

## *WHAT YOU NEED TO KNOW*
## *ABOUT YOUR PRESCRIPTIONS*

Certain things are important to know about each and every one of your prescribed medications. I suggest that you gather these answers from the interactions you have with both your physician and your pharmacist. You have the right to this information, and can expect that your care providers will be forthcoming with answers.

The Institute for Safe Medication Practices (ISMP), a ten-year-old nonprofit organization working to make the medication-use process less prone to errors and mistakes, suggests that you know the following prior to leaving the pharmacy.

Before you leave the pharmacy, your pharmacist should give you printed information about the medication and make sure that you understand the answers to these questions:

1. What are the brand and generic names of the medications?
2. What does it look like?
3. Why am I taking it?
4. How much should I take, and how often?
5. When is the best time to take it?
6. How long will I need to take it?
7. What side effects should I expect, and what should I do if they happen?
8. What should I do if I miss a dose?
9. Does this interact with my other medications or any foods?
10. Does this replace anything else I was taking?
11. Where and how do I store it?[5]

In addition, you can be an informed and active participant in your health care decisions, including the decision to take medications. In *FDA Consumer,* Bullman suggests three actions to help you in your drug-taking process:

1. Take part in your treatment decisions.
2. Follow your treatment plan.
3. Watch for problems and get help in solving them.[6]

These three items include participating in your health decision making, asking questions as needed, and continuing to work with your doctors and pharmacists to help solve problems that may arise. Bullman suggests that you need not be embarrassed about asking questions and following up with your caregivers.[7] You can help yourself to comply by being knowledgeable about the medications prescribed for you or a loved one.

# Chapter 2

# Why Compliance with Medications Is Important

When you see a physician for care of a disease or ailment, you are asked to do numerous things in order to become well again. Sometimes it is not possible to be 100 percent well, but each of us can be healthy within the health state in which we find ourselves. The prescribing of one or more medications is a common outcome of seeing a physician for care. Over 60 percent of office visits to physicians result in the prescribing of more than one medication per patient.[1] Drugs can provide an important opportunity to help you get well. In order to utilize medications appropriately, compliance with regimens is crucial for you and those for whom you provide care. Everybody seems to talk about compliance, but you have many chances to improve it for yourself and loved ones.

## *DEFINITIONS*

First, what is compliance? Compliance refers to how much of a prescribed dose that you actually take. Compliance is certainly not an either/or patient behavior; thus, the definitions of compliance behavior must be varied to reflect varying patient behaviors. The four types of compliance are (see also Figure 2.1)

1. initial noncompliance
2. partial compliance
3. complete compliance
4. hypercompliance

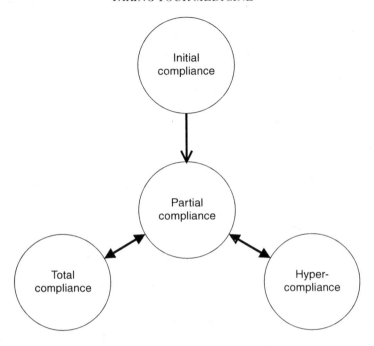

Initial compliance—Having your prescription filled at a pharmacy
Partial compliance—Taking some of your medication as prescribed
Complete compliance—Taking your medication exactly as prescribed
Hypercompliance—Taking too much of your medication

FIGURE 2.1. Interrelationship of various types of compliance. *Source:* Fincham JE, Wertheimer AI. Initial drug noncompliance in the elderly. *Journal of Geriatric Drug Therapy* 1986; 1(1):19-29.

*Initial noncompliance* occurs when you have a written prescription to be filled, or perhaps a prescription phoned in by a physician to your pharmacy, and you do not pick up the prescription or have it filled for whatever reason. Estimates suggest that 20 percent of all prescriptions written in the United States are never filled. Other studies have shown that ~30 percent of prescriptions are transmitted to a pharmacist without the patient knowing that this has happened.[2] So take heart, compliance mistakes are not always yours! Communication is sometimes lacking in our health care system.

Also, through the process of seeking care and deciding to self-treat, an individual may enter the health care system only so far—perhaps to obtain a diagnosis—but will not rely on a physician for treatment of the diagnosed condition. Self-help or self-care may be utilized to try to treat the condition.

*Partial compliance* occurs when you take your medication but not the full dosage or all the time. The average rate for this type of compliance is around 50 percent, but it varies from patient to patient and from time to time.

*Complete compliance* is the situation when you are 100 percent compliant 100 percent of the time. This is tough to do! It is admirable if you can reach this level of compliance, but you are not to be discouraged if you cannot reach it. You should try very hard to be as compliant as you can within your circumstances and particular health status.

*Hypercompliance* is when you take the medication over and above what is recommended or prescribed. This can be dangerous and detrimental to your health; be cautious about taking too much of anything, including your prescription medications.

---

**KEY POINT**

*Do not spend a lot of time placing yourself in one category or another regarding compliance, just promise yourself to do better and then follow through with efforts to improve.*

---

In Figure 2.1, you will notice that the arrows for some of the four segments are interconnected and go both ways. It may be that one form of compliance leads to another. Some people may be completely compliant with one medication and have trouble with other types. You may initially comply with a medication, begin to partially comply, and then totally comply with your medication regimen. This is the ultimate goal of your medication-taking activities. You should not proceed from partial compliance to hypercompliance, or taking too much of your medication. Taking medicine may be complex, and complying is difficult for some to achieve. So, from time to time each of these categories may pertain to you or a loved one.

## *WHY COMPLIANCE MATTERS*

So, what is the big deal with patient compliance? Why is so much attention paid to noncompliance and its ramifications? The reasons lie in the health, societal, and economic consequences of patient non-compliance. The effects of noncompliance can be felt from physician and patient to families and beyond. Noncompliance leads to treatment failure, the need for more health care services, lack of efficacy of drug regimens, and prolongation of a return to health.

The conglomeration of drug misuse, patient noncompliance, and adverse drug events are often lumped into the term *drug morbidity.* This refers to health-related problems that are directly due to not using drugs properly. In some cases, patients are noncompliant rather than openly disagreeing with their doctors. Noncompliance may seem to some patients a viable alternative to complying with drug therapy regimens, especially when a patient may have definite opposing viewpoints to those of a physician.

The effects of noncompliance can be costly for all involved. It has been estimated that the economic costs of patient drug misuse to tax-payers in the United States each year approach $100 billion.[3] What this means is that for every dollar that is spent on drugs in the health care system, another $1.33 is spent to deal with harmful effects from the misuse of these drugs. Further, it is estimated that the improper use of prescription drugs causes nearly 125,000 deaths per year and accounts for 19 percent of all hospital admissions in the United States alone.[4] However, please know that patient noncompliance does not account for all of the expenses or mortality alluded to here (in this case, deaths due to drug misuse), but it does account for a significant amount of harm. The amount of harm may vary, but it makes sense to always minimize problems with our health or health care treatment.

---

### KEY POINT

*Compliance with drugs you take now can save you money in the future, but more important, it can avoid other disease complications.*

---

Consider your own health care situation or that of family members. If you are hospitalized due to noncompliance with drugs that are prescribed for you, the "costs" you pay are significant. An adage says that for every day you spend in the hospital, it takes five days to recover from the stay once you are home again. This affects your ability to attend school, work, or other necessary activities, which in turn leads to lower grades, loss of wages, out-of-pocket expenses, and perhaps further necessary drug therapies.

Consider the following scenario. Say you have diabetes mellitus (high blood sugar). There are two forms of diabetes: juvenile (Type I) and adult onset (Type II).[5] Basically, one form develops in childhood or adolescence and the other occurs when a person is an adult. In the early stages of Type II diabetes, many people's conditions can be controlled through nutrition, diet, and use of oral hypoglycemic agents. These agents include drugs such as

- Actos (pioglitazone),
- Avandia (rosiglitazone),
- Glyset (miglitol),
- Precose (acarbose),
- Glucophage (metformin),
- Prandin (repaglinide),
- Amaryl (glimepiride), and
- DiaBeta, Glynase, or Micronase (all brand names for glyburide)

If a Type II diabetic patient does not comply with the prescribed regimen for these drugs, other problems related to diabetes may occur. The patient may be required to take other drugs, administer insulin shots, or wear an insulin pump. The long-term consequences of untreated or undertreated diabetes may include such diseases or complications as

- kidney disease,
- blindness,
- cardiac problems,
- neurological damage,
- foot sores, or
- amputation.[6]

Noncompliance can also lead to further complications in other disease conditions, such as high blood pressure (hypertension). These might include

- arrhythmias,
- stroke,
- heart attack,
- heart failure,
- kidney disease, or
- cerebral or aortic aneurysms.[7]

Perhaps all that the patient needed to do to avoid these complications was to be compliant with one drug. Hypertension is becoming increasingly more common in the United States. A recent article estimated that one-third of all Americans over the age of eighteen have high blood pressure.[8] However, the rate of compliance with hypertensive drugs is estimated to be only 40 percent on average.

Other conditions are adversely affected by noncompliance with prescribed drugs. For example, the rate of compliance for persons with epilepsy taking therapy is 30 to 50 percent; for arthritic patients it is 55 to 71 percent; and for those taking lipid-lowering drugs (for high cholesterol) it is 17 percent. The consequences for noncompliance with epilepsy treatment may result in an increase in seizures; for the arthritic patient it may be a worsening of the condition; and for the person with a lipid disorder it may result in heart attack, stroke, or other cardiovascular and/or cerebrovascular problems.

In addition, it costs money to be put on other medications to treat conditions resulting from noncompliance with prescribed medications. The additional medications may be costly and certainly are avoidable.

You or a loved one may also lose productivity at work due to "presenteeism." This occurs when you are physically at work, but because of a physical or mental symptom or disease you are not optimally productive at your job. You are physically at work so to speak, but yet you are not there at 100 percent of your capabilities. You simply may be mentally not ready or able to be at work. This may occur with depression, upper respiratory tract infections, diabetes, or gastrointestinal disturbances. Each of these conditions is treatable with medications, but if noncompliance occurs, the patient may not be fully able to work.

Other costs may include lost wages, lost productivity, lost opportunity to influence the course of a disease in early stages, and the cost of time spent seeking further treatment from the same or new health care providers. If you are looking after an elderly family member, drug problems are a cause of admissions to long-term care (LTC) facilities. In fact, only 5 percent of the elderly reside in LTCs, but 25 percent of LTC residents are there because they cannot manage their medications on their own. Noncompliance is estimated to account for 45 percent of the drug-related problems that result in LTC admissions. It should be obvious that the costs associated with admitting a loved one to a nursing home are extensive. Other institutional expenses as a result of noncompliance can be costly, too. These scenarios may include emergency room (ER) visits or hospitalizations due to asthma or diabetes.

## *RISKS VERSUS BENEFITS*

As with any health care decision, there are risks and benefits associated with drug compliance. You may decide that the side effects that accompany a drug therapy are not worth the health benefit it offers. If you are prescribed a diuretic (e.g., hydrochlorothiazide, furosemide) to treat mild high blood pressure, you might decide that the effects of frequent urination, interruption of sleep to go to the bathroom, dizziness, drowsiness, and/or headache may not be worth putting up with. After all, for the most part, high blood pressure does not have any outward symptoms, but the cure might. Before opting out of all medication treatments, it might be worth talking with your doctor about other treatments that can help your blood pressure without the side effects mentioned here. Other options may exist; be sure to ask about them for chronic conditions such as high blood pressure, diabetes, asthma, high cholesterol, or high triglycerides. You might find that another therapy can work as well and cause you less trouble in the long run. You can certainly ask your pharmacist for options that can be recommended to your doctors as alternate therapies. In some cases, unpleasant effects can be mitigated by altering the dosage or the time of administration.

## IS 100 PERCENT COMPLIANCE
## ALWAYS NECESSARY?

Since I have already mentioned that it is difficult to be 100 percent compliant, how compliant must you be in order to control symptoms? This varies a great deal based on the particular drug, the disease that it treats, and the margin of error for not being compliant. If you are taking a birth-control pill to avoid pregnancy, a 100 percent rate of compliance is what you should aim for. However, if you forget to take a dose of the birth-control pill, taking two the next day can suffice. If you miss more than one day, you will need to use an alternate form of birth control until you can find out from your physician what you should do to resume the daily doses.

Also, if you have been prescribed an antibiotic to treat an infection, 100 percent compliance is what you should be trying to achieve. It is often the case that, after taking an antibiotic for a few days, we begin to feel better. Even though you might feel better, it is important to take the full course of the antibiotic. Your symptoms may improve after a few doses, but the underlying infection needs to be treated for the full course of time in order to eliminate as many bacteria as possible. I am as guilty as anyone with regard to antibiotics; it becomes difficult to complete the full therapy when you feel better and gain strength and energy. In some instances, you should take the forgotten dose as soon as you remember. However, just to be safe, always check with your doctor or pharmacist to be sure. Avoid at all costs doubling up on doses to get better twice as fast. *Do not* take a ten-day course of therapy in five days to hurry the healing process. You may end up with more problems than you bargained for.

Other chronic disease medications may be consumed at less than 100 percent and still achieve the intended therapeutic effect. Some would say that if you are compliant with 80 percent of your high blood pressure medications you should be okay. However, this depends to a great extent on the type of medication, the frequency of administration, and the severity of your hypertension. Also, if you have been prescribed a drug to be taken once daily for hypertension or heart failure, missing a day's dose can lead to problems.

If you take a medication for arthritis, skipping a dose will not hurt you. However, you will run into problems if you take the doses very sporadically and miss numerous doses. Your symptoms may reappear or you will notice that the drug does not seem to work as it once did. Or, if you take too many you may run into side effects with the medication, and be forced to take another medication to deal with the stomach problems.

A person with diabetes who is required to use insulin will suffer if doses are skipped or are not faithfully administered. Diabetics more so than many patients have specific needs as they pertain to control of blood-sugar levels. Often patients have to juggle diet, exercise, and insulin administration in order to control the disease and subsequent symptoms.

One of the great problem areas with regard to drug taking, regards the directions "take as necessary" or "take as needed." How much is necessary and how much is needed may seem perfectly clear to your doctor, but murky to you. If you are taking a drug to treat minor symptoms, such as allergies, nasal stuffiness, or congestion, you can judge for yourself how best to control symptoms. If it is a chronic condition, such as diabetes, hypertension, or epilepsy, the directions "take as needed" are simply not good enough for you to adequately know what to do with the medications, and you should ask your doctor or pharmacist to give clear instructions.

External creams or ointments to treat serious conditions may need to be used with 100 percent compliance, unless it is for a symptom that responds to intermittent therapy, in which case missing a dose will not cause you a great deal of grief. If you are to apply an external preparation to treat skin cancer, your compliance needs to approach or meet 100 percent. If you are being treated for poison ivy or poison oak, you may be able to skip a dose or two, although your symptoms may return quickly. A vaginal cream should be used for the full term; yeast infections can be tricky to treat and difficult to eliminate if the full dose is not inserted. Topical creams and ointments to treat skin rashes may clear the condition quickly, and you may not need to use all the product that is prescribed. External ointments and creams have shelf lives assigned, just as any other prescription medications. Be sure you know the expiration date for the product and discard it when this time arrives. If the product is for symptomatic relief, you may be able to use the product numerous times in the future without concern. In this instance, hang on to the product and do not discard it; this may save you time and money down the road. How do you know if it is okay to save it? Always check with your health care providers to be sure.

If you think that you are at risk for compliance problems but are not sure, ask yourself these questions and let your caregivers know your responses:

1. Do I miss doses of my medication all the time?
2. Do I frequently miss a dose of my medication?
3. Do I sometimes miss a dose of my medication?
4. Do I rarely miss doses of my medications?
5. Do I never miss any of my scheduled doses?

For which of these questions was your answer "yes"? Think about how you can change behaviors if you see yourself in the first three categories. Above all else, let others know where you fall regarding these questions, and ask them to help you if you need assistance.

In summary, the more we examine compliance, the more complex it becomes. You should try to be as compliant as you can to avoid additional costs and burdens of disease. We all are noncompliant at one time or another, but it is important to achieve the best levels of compliance possible. Do not worry about your past behavior, just try to do the very best that you can starting now. If you need help in being compliant, be thankful that you can recognize this and then obtain help to improve your compliance. It is not possible to be 100 percent with every drug that is prescribed for you. As noted previously, some therapies require you to be 100 percent compliant; in other cases, coming close to 100 percent is acceptable to control symptoms and diseases. If you are unsure about your target level of compliance, ask your pharmacist or physician to guide you through your various medications to pinpoint those you need to be 100 percent compliant with and those that you can come close to and not suffer too badly. If you can improve your compliance rates, help control symptoms, and achieve goals consider yourself a star; this is tough to do and worthy of praise if you can pull it off!

Compliance is important now, and will no doubt remain an important issue for years to come. A lot rides on the ability of individuals to follow through on medications prescribed for them. Stakeholders in the enhancing of compliance include health practitioners (physicians, pharmacists, nurses, etc.), health system institutions (hospitals, long-term care facilities, other institutions), insurers, payers (employers), government agencies such as the CMS (Centers for Medicare & Medicaid Services), and—most important of all—you, the patient.

---

**KEY POINT**

*Noncompliance affects many persons and components of the health care system. Do whatever you can to help yourself comply better.*

---

This issue is of such importance that it has been suggested that oversight of providers to ensure their patients' compliance may be commonplace in the future.[9] Whether this will happen is debatable. What is not at issue is that compliance saves time and expense over the long run. Appropriate compliance with medications allows patients and providers to better achieve therapeutic goals. This in turn enables patients to enjoy better self-care, more appropriately medicate themselves and loved ones, and thus avoid other costly forms of health care services. The final endpoint is that patients can remain in the optimum level of health for them as individuals.

# Chapter 3

# How to Choose a Pharmacist

We often spend a great deal of time selecting the right person to take care of many of our needs. We may ask about mechanics, home repair persons, security consultants, and others that perform important functions in our lives. You should spend a similar amount of time selecting an important health care professional, such as your pharmacist. Outside of your physicians, your pharmacist can provide you with more significant therapeutic drug information than any other health professional. Thus, it is important to choose your pharmacist well and examine what is important to you as a patient seeking care from a pharmacist.

## *PROFESSIONALISM AND ACCESSIBILITY*

### *What Body Language Tells You*

It is said that when we communicate, 95 percent of what is transmitted is nonverbal.[1] You can tell a great deal about people and their responsiveness to you from their body language or nonverbal communication. If your pharmacist does not look you in the eye when speaking to you, has his or her arms crossed or stands in a slouched position, it may be difficult for you to know whether you are speaking to a receptive individual. A professional pharmacist should always make eye contact with you, lean toward you when speaking to you, and convey to you that you are an important person. The manner in which a person looks at you and his or her facial expression indicates whether he or she respects you. In addition, a professional individual always dresses appropriately. Clean clothes and appropriate personal hygiene speak volumes to you without the individual saying a word. Pay close attention to how your pharmacists communicate with you, the clothes that they are wearing, and the cleanliness of the individuals and the pharmacy itself. Through the process of evaluating these and other attributes of the pharmacist and the pharmacy, can you place faith in the individual?

A word of caution is in order: you cannot always tell just by looks or demeanor. Robert Courtney, a Kansas City, Missouri, pharmacist, was charged by grand jury indictment, on August 23, 2001, with eight counts of tampering with a consumer product, six counts of adulteration of a drug, and six counts of misbranding of a drug. He was subsequently sentenced to 360 months in federal prison.[2] In a case that drew national attention, Courtney pleaded guilty to diluting chemotherapy and other drugs at his Kansas City pharmacy. His plea agreement recommended a sentence of seventeen to twenty-two years, but a federal district judge imposed a longer sentence. Robert Courtney by all accounts was dressed professionally and was looked up to and admired by his patients. Look at other factors as well when you choose your pharmacist; a lot is riding on your choice.

Counterfeiting of prescription drugs was unheard of just a few years ago; unfortunately it is now a commonly discussed issue. Recent FBI arrests have highlighted the current problems with the counterfeiting of prescription drugs.[3] FBI agents made more arrests in September 2004 in an operation to dismantle a ring believed to be responsible for trafficking over $56 million in stolen and counterfeit pharmaceuticals over the previous fifteen months. Pharmacists were implicated in this operation, so you have to find a pharmacist you can trust, and monitor to assure the trust is well placed.

Appropriate communication style (both verbal and nonverbal), cleanliness, and respectful demeanor will not always guarantee that your pharmacist will act professionally and ethically, but they can be used to guide your decision. Other factors should be considered, but use your own intuition about the first impression that the pharmacist is making. Do you feel that you can place the care of yourself or your loved ones in this person's hands?

### Is the Pharmacist Accessible?

Your pharmacist should be readily accessible to you for your needs concerning the medications that you or a loved one is taking. Your pharmacist can be a valuable source of information about drugs, their effects, and proper usage. You should be comfortable asking your pharmacist about side effects, adverse reactions, and expectations for your drug therapy. Pharmacists are the most accessible health professionals, and you should use this to the fullest extent possible. No one in the health care system is as knowledgeable about drugs and as approachable in the practice setting.

Your pharmacist should be available to answer a question at any time about the medications you currently take or are considering taking. If you are unsure who you are speaking with at the pharmacy, ask to speak with the pharmacist. If the pharmacist is unable to talk right then, set a time to talk later about your questions and concerns.

It may be that you can speak with the pharmacist on the phone and receive the answers that you seek. Pharmacists are very accustomed to speaking with doctors, nurses, and patients on the phone. It is commonplace and a good way for you to ensure privacy and obtain the needed information. You may have more time to talk on the phone with the pharmacist than in a face-to-face scenario. Find out what works best for you and your needs, and follow through to find the answers you are seeking.

## KNOWLEDGE AND REPUTATION

### Concerns About Certain Medications When Caring for an Elderly Individual

If you are caring for an elderly family member, you should know that drug use in the elderly is fraught with difficulty. A recent article in *The New York Times* reviewed an alarming study of drug prescribing for the elderly conducted by the Duke Clinical Research Institute.[4] The study found that 20 percent of the elderly had been prescribed at least one unsafe drug, 15 percent had been prescribed two, and 4 percent had received three unsafe drugs. These drugs had the potential to cause serious drug reactions in the seniors receiving them. Elsewhere, researchers have compiled a list of sixty-six drugs considered unsafe for use in the elderly.[5] Make sure that the pharmacist caring for your senior loved one is knowledgeable about this list and the drugs that are chronicled and can supply you with alternate suggestions for treatment. Numerous sources present this information, and your pharmacist will know where to look in order to obtain it.

## Referrals from Friends

One source of information about pharmacies is the counsel of your friends and acquaintances. If someone you know has had good luck with a pharmacy, chances are good that you will as well. Check with people you know well and trust: How are they treated at the pharmacy? Do they feel comfortable recommending their pharmacist to you? Are the services that they receive equally important to you? Do they trust their pharmacist and pharmacy to take care of all their medication needs?

If you are new to an area, ask neighbors or co-workers which physicians or pharmacists they use for their health needs. If you have been referred to a specialist for care, ask your referring physician who he or she would go to first for health needs. Perhaps asking a nurse in your doctor's office for information can be an option as well.

## HONESTY AND ETHICAL BEHAVIOR

### How You Can Spot Dishonesty

If your pharmacist refuses to transfer your prescription to another pharmacy, demand that it be done. Some prescriptions cannot be transferred or switched from one pharmacy to another; these include Schedule II prescriptions (e.g., drugs such Percodan, OxyContin, Vicodin). However, your prescriptions belong to you, and you can have your records transferred to another pharmacy any time you wish. If you have remaining refills on prescriptions and are told that you cannot transfer the prescription to another pharmacy, you are being treated dishonestly. If the pharmacist continues to refuse to transfer your records to the pharmacy of your choice, the pharmacist at the new pharmacy you wish to frequent can call your physician and obtain new prescriptions for you. You are free to have your prescriptions filled and refilled at the pharmacy of your choosing. This is your right as a patient and not subject to the whims of the pharmacist.

## *What to Do if Your Pharmacist's Behavior Is Questionable*

If you suspect substandard care is being provided to you or, worse yet, you are being treated dishonestly, I encourage you to ask for help from another pharmacist. If you cannot obtain any satisfaction from your current pharmacist, ask your friends or family for the name of a pharmacist who takes care of them. You can also ask your physician or another health care professional in the doctor's office for the name of a recommended pharmacist. I also recommend that you contact the state board of pharmacy where you live and register a complaint if you suspect dishonesty on the part of the pharmacist. Chances are that if this is happening to you, it is happening to others as well. You need to take the step of contacting someone to see if something can be done about the pharmacist or pharmacy.

## *Tips to Spot an Unethical Pharmacist*

As much as we would like to believe that all pharmacists are ethical and carry out their responsibilities in an aboveboard fashion, some pharmacists are not ethical. What follows are some things to consider that indicate unprofessional behavior on the part of a pharmacist.

### *Background*

Pharmacists hold a special role in the health care system, and accompanying this role is a tremendous responsibility to practice the profession of pharmacy in a completely ethical and moral manner. However, pharmacists may not be ethical, so the following are some indications of unprofessional behavior on the part of a pharmacist. How many are unethical is a question that cannot be answered. One is too many. Protect yourself and your family by evaluating the pharmacists that provide care to you, and consider several items when viewing the appropriateness of care provided to you and yours. I hope none of the following has happened or is happening to you, but if it is you need to protect your rights and receive the proper care you deserve.

*Counseling When Obtaining New Prescriptions*

U.S. federal law and subsequent state rules and regulations require that you be offered counseling on prescriptions that you have filled. These federal regulations (Omnibus Budget Reconciliation Act of 1990 [OBRA '90]) were initially applicable to patients receiving care through the various state Medicaid assistance programs; however, all states have now passed regulations that expand this requirement to all patients. The offer to counsel means just that—you should be asked if you would like to hear information about your medications. In practice what happens is that you are asked to sign a log thrust in front of you that says you have declined the offer to receive counseling. Many people think this signature log simply indicates that they have picked up a prescription, but this is not the case. You should be told what this signature form means and asked if you would care to learn about the drugs that you are receiving. The letter of the law is being met by the signature log, but this does not fulfill the pharmacist's obligation to counsel you if you would like to receive further information.

It is unethical for a pharmacist to refuse to speak with you about your medications. Insist that you receive instructions on proper use of the drugs prescribed and dispensed to you. If for some reason it is not convenient for the pharmacist to fully counsel you when you pick up a prescription, find a time in your schedule when it would be convenient for you to speak with the pharmacist by phone, if necessary.

If you happen to use a mail-order pharmacy for your prescriptions, the mail-order pharmacy must provide you with a toll-free number to call for questions about the medications you receive. You deserve to receive full information about medications that you take regardless of how you obtain the drugs—by mail, in person, via delivery, or through someone picking up your medications and bringing them to you.

You do not need to wait until you have a prescription filled before asking a pharmacist about your medications. You can call and speak to your pharmacist at any time. Also, you can speak to a pharmacist if you happen to be in the pharmacy and have a question. A pharmacist should always be available to answer your questions, whether you happen to be a patient at that pharmacy or not. Virtually every pharmacist will assist you with answering questions, regardless of where you obtain your medications.

---
**KEY POINT**

*Although occasionally it is expected that your pharmacist may be too busy to speak with you, if you consistently have trouble when trying to speak with him or her, consider finding a new pharmacy.*

---

*Proper Dispensing*

Guidelines govern the type of medication that you are dispensed after your physician writes or phones in prescriptions to a pharmacy for filling. Depending on the drug in question, a prescription might specify a brand-name product only, or it may allow a generic substitute for the brand-name product, which will save you money.

---
**KEY POINT**

*In order to save you money, your physician may write a prescription for a generic medication. Your pharmacist may also generically substitute in order to save you money.*

---

*Brand-Name and Generic Drugs*

Several possible types of drugs can be dispensed for you as a patient. A drug may be available as only a brand-name product. When a drug is first on the market, no generic option is available to you. In this case, the product still has patent protection, the duration of which depends on the amount of time it took for the drug to reach the market after going through the phases of approval required by the FDA. A generic drug may also be referred to as a multisource product, meaning that several manufacturers make that drug.

---
**KEY POINT**

*Generic substitutes are available for some but not all brand-name prescription drugs. Ask your pharmacist if a generic is available for your prescription; it will save you money.*

---

You can give a pharmacist the benefit of the doubt if you suspect an error is being made regarding generic or brand-name drugs, but prod and push to find out exactly what is occurring. If you are dispensed a generic alternative for your prescription, you should pay the generic price and not be charged for the brand-name product. If you refill a prescription and receive a generic alternative but pay the same amount as when you obtained a brand-name product, you are being deceived by the pharmacist. You should always be told when a generic substitute is provided to you and informed about the cost savings between the brand-name version and the generic version. The whole point of using a generic product is to save the consumer money, not increase the profits for the pharmacy. If you feel that you are paying too much, challenge the pharmacist and find out exactly what you are paying for, as well as the savings you are receiving in comparison to the brand-name version of the product.

Also, if the prescription label indicates the prescription was filled with a brand-name product but the drugs in the container are generics, you are being deceived and your prescription is mislabeled. Mislabeling is a violation of pharmacy practice acts in every state. A pharmacist cannot fill a brand-name–labeled container with a generic alternative. Challenge the pharmacist if this occurs: the prescription may have been filled in error, or perhaps the wrong drug is being dispensed to you.

Your state board of pharmacy should be notified if either of the following scenarios is occurring:

1. You are receiving a generic substitute but are being charged the same price as the brand-name product.
2. Your prescription label indicates that you are receiving the brand-name version of a drug product but the prescription is being filled with the generic version of the drug.

If you still feel that you are not receiving satisfaction, you can enlist the services of an attorney—I hope this never happens to you, but if it does, do not feel intimidated by seeking legal help. If you cannot afford the services of an attorney, legal aid services are available for those who cannot pay for costly legal assistance. If you do not know of such a clinic, you can contact a law school in your area. Simply call the main number to the school and ask if they are aware of any legal aid clinics in the area that can help you with a health care professional issue. Most law schools have clinics for varying groups, but a contact at a local law school would certainly know about other resources in the area.

## Shorting the Amounts but Charging the Full Price

Be aware of the amount of the drug that is dispensed to you and the amount specified on the label. If the label indicates 100 tablets and you are receiving less, challenge the pharmacist to give you the full amount. If you see a pattern of charging you full prices for less-than-labeled amounts, you are receiving unethical care from your pharmacist.

## Charging for Services

If you are being charged extra for services over and above what you are paying for prescriptions and have not agreed to purchase extra services, you are probably being overcharged. A pharmacist may provide expanded services for you, services for which you have agreed to pay, and there is nothing wrong with this. However, if you are being charged for the pharmacist to contact your physician or insurance company on your behalf, you are being overcharged. If you are being told that you have to pay a membership fee in order to obtain services, you are being unethically treated. If you have a certain type of insurance and are told by the pharmacist that you will have to pay extra in order to receive care, this is wrong. If you are told that you have to pay extra because you are asking to have your prescriptions transferred to another pharmacy, this is deceitful, unethical conduct on the part of the pharmacist.

## Bait and Switch

If after checking on a comparative price for a prescription you are charged a greater amount, you are being treated unfairly. This could conceivably occur with a new prescription filled either with a brand-name product or a generic substitute. Also, if you pay one price the first time you have a prescription filled but the subsequent refills are much more costly, ask why. Price increases are commonplace in the prescription drug market; just make sure that what you are paying is indeed what you should be paying. There is nothing wrong with double-checking to make sure that you are being charged the correct amount.

## Refusal to Fill Your Prescription

A pharmacist may choose not to fill your prescription. That is a right that pharmacists have in some cases. Some pharmacists choose to not compound prescriptions from basic ingredients to make creams, ointments, or some liquid preparations. Some pharmacies do not participate in specific drug benefit plans. Pharmacists are not required to participate in all plans available to consumers. In fact, some plans may exclude certain pharmacies from participating.

However, it is not legal for a pharmacist to refuse to fill a prescription because of your personal characteristics. Nor is it legal to fill only certain prescriptions for certain individuals and not for others, even though they both have the same drug coverage. A pharmacist cannot choose to fill some prescriptions for you because they are profitable and not to fill others due to a low profit margin. If you have insurance coverage for prescription drugs and the drug you are seeking is covered under your insurance policy, the pharmacist should fill your prescription.

In several recent instances, there have been cases of pharmacists refusing to fill prescriptions based on their religious convictions,[6] for instance, pharmacists who did not fill prescriptions for birth-control pills. Pharmacists have also refused to fill emergency contraception prescriptions for high-dose combinations of birth-control pills. I personally feel these actions are unprofessional on the part of the pharmacists in question. I can understand a situation in which a pharmacist may defer filling a prescription to an associate that is on duty at the same time; however, to leave a patient stranded without recourse is inexcusable. This is my opinion, based on my beliefs and practice experience as a pharmacist.

However, there are instances when it is professionally justifiable to not fill a prescription for a patient. If a pharmacist refuses to fill a prescription due to the danger of a drug interaction with other medications you are taking, or it appears that there is an error on the part of the physician in prescribing a certain medication, these are certainly good reasons for not filling the prescription. If there appears to be overuse of certain drugs or a previous documented intolerance to a drug or a class of drugs, these are also good reasons for not filling a prescription. In these cases, the pharmacist is serving as the patient's advocate, not placing a judgment on the patient. I see a need for this patient advocacy for therapeutic reasons, but cannot see the judgment role by a pharmacist for religious reasons as being acceptable.

## Furnishing You with the Best Price Available

Always find out how much you are "saving" when you obtain a "special" price on a prescription. If you are receiving a generic substitute, find out how much the savings are. If a generic drug is available for your prescription, find out if you are eligible to receive this. If you pay a copayment for your prescriptions, find out how to best maximize this. If, for example, you can obtain several months supply of a maintenance medication and pay just one copayment, you will save money. To find the answers to these questions, ask your pharmacist or call several pharmacies.

## Drugs and Expiration (Freshness) Dating

All drugs are required to have a manufacturer-supplied expiration date for each prescription medication marketed in the United States. Pharmacies routinely check for outdated products and have mechanisms to return the product to the manufacturer for replacements or refunds. Most medications when dispensed have, as a rule, an expiration date that is listed as one year from the date the prescription was filled. However, you may be dispensed a drug with a shorter shelf life, and if this is the case, the one-year rule does not apply. You will not know what the original expiration date is unless you ask the pharmacist. Make sure that the drugs that you are receiving are in date and correctly marked. Some items, such as ophthalmic (for use in the eyes) or otic (for use in the ears) preparations, have a shorter expiration date due to the way the items are used. For any ophthalmic preparation, I recommend that you discard the remaining amount after ninety days. You may not have to use the product for this length of time, anyway. The tube or ointment may have an extended expiration date listed somewhere on the product itself, but please note that once the sterile seal is broken this expiration date is invalid. The expiration date put on these containers by the manufacturer assumes that the product is unopened and thus remains sterile; once opened the sterility is lost and the shelf life becomes shorter.

## Transferring Prescriptions from One Pharmacy to Another

It is always possible to transfer your prescription from one pharmacy to another. This assumes, of course, that the prescription in question has refills remaining. Prescriptions that are not refillable, those with no refills remaining, or certain categories of prescriptions (e.g., scheduled drugs, such as some pain medications and/or sleep aids) are not eligible to be transferred from one pharmacy to another. If you have your prescriptions filled at a chain pharmacy, the prescriptions can easily be transferred from one chain pharmacy location to another. This can be very handy when traveling out of state. Prescriptions filled at mail-order pharmacies or local community pharmacies can also be transferred from one pharmacy to another. Do not believe a pharmacist who tells you that a prescription with refills remaining cannot be transferred from the original pharmacy to another pharmacy.

## Who Owns Your Prescription?

When you have a prescription filled, the pharmacy by state law must retain the paper copy of the prescription. The same holds true when a physician will phone a prescription in to a pharmacy for you. Having said this, you do have rights pertaining to your prescriptions. As previously noted, you do have the right to have your refillable prescriptions transferred from one pharmacy to another. Pharmacies must do this if you request it. You should be able to obtain a record of the prescriptions that you have had filled at any time. Pharmacies should willingly provide this information to you; if they do not do so, they are acting in an unethical manner.

## Privacy and Respect

Regulations (described in Chapter 6) stipulate that you have a right to privacy regarding the records of medical care provided to you and loved ones. This certainly pertains to prescription drug information about you and your family as well. This information cannot be shared with anyone without your explicit approval. Make sure you ensure this is being followed by informing the pharmacist who fills your prescriptions that you do not want your pharmacy records shared with anyone outside of the pharmacy.

You deserve to be treated with respect in a pharmacy. You are entitled to receive counseling from the pharmacist each and every time you have a prescription filled or stop at the pharmacy to ask a question. Consultations with the pharmacist should be accomplished in a quiet, private area of the pharmacy or close to it. If you do not feel comfortable with the surroundings when speaking with the pharmacist, ask to move to a more private area. By all means avoid a situation in a larger store where a clerk blares over a loudspeaker: "Prescription ready for John Thomason" or, worse yet, "Paxil prescription ready for Luke Mathias." The former is less severe than the latter; however, both are inappropriate. Also, around the pharmacy counter itself, do not let a situation occur as follows: "Pharmacist Jones, Mr. Delgado has a question about his AIDS medication regimen." If Pharmacist Jones can hear this request, anybody else in earshot can hear as well. All of these situations are unethical. You should not hesitate to choose another pharmacy if this happens to you, and report the occurrence to the state board of pharmacy in your area.

## The People Behind the Front Counter

Behind the front counter in a retail pharmacy is the area where your prescriptions are filled. It is likely that individuals who are not pharmacists will be there. Pharmacy technicians are ancillary helpers who can do some of the tasks required to complete a prescription order. Technicians are allowed to retrieve bulk bottles from shelving, count the correct number of units called for on the prescription, and prepare a prescription label. In some states they are allowed to place a prescription label on the container; in other states they are prohibited from doing so—only the pharmacist can do this. Technicians can also prepare compounded prescriptions and intravenous (IV) preparations. The pharmacist on duty at the time of these activities then checks the work of the technician for accuracy and completeness and completes the preparation of the prescription order. Varying ratios occur between states concerning how many technicians can be monitored by one pharmacist. There might be a variance from a 1:1 technician-to-pharmacist ratio to a 2:1, 3:1, or 4:1 ratio allowed by pharmacy rules and regulations.

Other individuals may not work on prescription orders in a pharmacy. Clerks, delivery persons, or other employees are not allowed to participate in the filling of prescriptions in any state. If you suspect that this is occurring with your prescriptions, contact the board of pharmacy and alert the pharmacist about these activities. No one other than a pharmacist or a technician is allowed to participate in the completion of a prescription order. A pharmacist must also be present in the pharmacy when prescription orders are completed and dispensed to you.

Many states now require that pharmacists and pharmacy technicians wear badges that indicate their status as either a pharmacist or a technician. If you cannot ascertain who is filling your prescriptions by observation, ask probing questions until you find out who is completing your prescription orders. If in fact a nonprofessional is filling your prescription or preparing ingredients for your prescriptions, contact the pharmacist in charge (they all are required to have an individual so named) and register a complaint. Also, contact the state board of pharmacy in your area and file a complaint against the pharmacy.

In several of the previous scenarios, I have encouraged you to be proactive regarding the prescriptions that you have filled and monitoring your pharmacy for ethical and appropriate behavior. Virtually all pharmacies operate in an aboveboard and ethical fashion in treating patients. However, since there are some who are not ethical and are breaking the law, they should be identified and reported. This is not only for your sake, but for the well-being of future patients in pharmacies. State boards of pharmacy are put in place to protect the health of the public; they are not created to protect pharmacies. Thus, you should consider boards of pharmacy to be in fact "consumer protection" agencies for your and your family's medication, health, and well-being. If your state board of pharmacy does not appear to be responsive to your requests or concerns, contact the attorney general's office in your state.

### *Where to Report Dishonesty or Substandard Care*

Because of concerns over liability, one health care professional will rarely speak negatively about another. A physician will not speak disparagingly of another doctor; pharmacists are reluctant to say negative things about other pharmacists. If you have serious concerns about a pharmacist, you can seek help from state boards of medical practice or state boards of pharmacy. Each practitioner is expected to have a current license in the state where he or she is providing care. State boards of pharmacy and medical examiners all have mechanisms for you to report poor care or mistreatment. In the case of pharmacy, you can access individual state boards of pharmacy Web sites through <www.napb.net> by clicking on "Who We Are" and then clicking on "Boards of Pharmacy." Contact information is listed for each state board of pharmacy. Each state presents information a little differently, but you can access information about the pharmacist in question, his or her license number, and information on how you can report problem pharmacists or pharmacies.

State boards of medical examiners have similar Web sites for each individual state. Their Web address through the Federation of State Medical Boards is as follows: <www.fsmb.org/members.htm>. On this site you can click on the state of interest and, by following linkages on each individual state medical board home page, access the information on how to file a complaint regarding the medical care that you have been provided.

In either case, you will be required to furnish information that may include

1. your name, address, and contact information;
2. the physician or pharmacist in question;
3. the license number of the practitioner in question;
4. the date and time that you received care; and
5. specific, detailed information about why you are filing the complaint.

You may also receive instructions about follow-up procedures that may be necessary after you file the complaint. This is a last-resort option should you not be able to receive satisfactory resolution of the issue with the individual pharmacist, physician, or other pertinent person in authority.


## WHEN YOU CANNOT CHOOSE YOUR PHARMACY

Your insurance coverage may mandate which pharmacy(ies) you may use. In this case, you may have to use a mail-service pharmacy in order to receive coverage for your prescriptions. If so, you can still request certain things from your pharmacist and demand that you receive them. If you have questions and need to speak with a pharmacist, insist that you be able to speak with one when you call the toll-free number or request that a pharmacist phone you at a mutually agreeable time.

If you need to have the pharmacy contact your physician, a mail-service pharmacy can do this as well. Try to obtain the best service that you can. If for some reason the service falls short, demand other options or let your insurance company know that you have complaints, and be specific about what your expectations are and how they are not being met.


## OTHER SERVICES

It will be useful to make a list of services that are important to you. Does the pharmacy deliver medications to customers' homes? Do they charge for such services? Can you fill prescriptions after hours? This may not be so important for new prescriptions, but it certainly is for refills. Many chain community pharmacies and/or food market pharmacies now have extended hours of operation, even twenty-four-hour service, so you know that you can obtain prescriptions most anytime. However, even with twenty-four-hour operations it may be difficult to fill a prescription sometimes, say on a holiday. Will there be someone who can fill your prescriptions on an emergency basis? Many independent community pharmacies will not have pharmacies open for twenty-four hours a day, but will open the pharmacy for emergencies. This may be important if you care for young children. Children seem to get sick more often than not when it is late at night or very early in the morning.

Because of changes in insurance coverage and specifications, you may need to have prescription medications approved before they can be dispensed. This is usually the case with most pharmacy benefit management (PBM) companies, who make decisions about which drugs are covered under their plans. If your medication is not one of the drugs on your PBM's list, you will need what is termed "prior approval" before it can be filled. Your pharmacy can anticipate this need, contact the PBM ahead of time, and have your prescriptions ready to be filled when you need them. This is an extra, customer-focused service that will save you time, and if your pharmacy provides this service, it will be very useful. These types of value-added services help you realize you have made the correct choice regarding your pharmacy; if you do not have such service provided to you, you may wish to seek another pharmacy to meet you and your family's needs.

These and other services may be very important to you and your family, so spend extra time choosing the pharmacist to meet your needs. By all means, if you find your care is below standard, find another pharmacy to serve you better.

The bottom line is that you must be able to trust those who provide care to you and those you care for. Once thought impenetrable, the safety net of prescription distribution in the United States has been found to be "full of holes".[7] Pharmacists have been implicated in the counterfeiting and illegal distribution of fake drugs. If you do not trust those who care for you, you will not get well as quickly as you would with health professionals that you do trust. Quality, value, service, and technology, even if they are provided in an exemplary fashion, are not worth much if you cannot place trust in the providers of your health care. Trust is very important in many components of our life; it is the crucial element in your relationships with all your health care providers—physicians, pharmacists, optometrists, podiatrists, nurses, occupational therapists, or physical therapists.

# Chapter 4

# What the Doctor or Pharmacist Needs to Know About Your Health

As a general rule, the more information your health providers know about you and your health, the better care they can provide and the better off you will be. If your pharmacist offers to help you with remembering to take your medicine, do not be embarrassed or ashamed of having trouble remembering.

It is now commonplace for us to see multiple physicians. We might see a general practitioner and be referred to a specialist such as an internist, a cardiologist, an endocrinologist, an oncologist, or others. Each of these physicians needs to know what the other physicians are prescribing for you.

The more accurate the information you provide your physician about your health history, the more accurate your medical records will be. As the quality of your records increases, so will the quality of the medical care that you receive.

## MEDICAL CONDITIONS

Each of your care providers, or the providers of care for your family members, needs to understand all of the medical conditions for which you have been treated in the past. You can request that your medical records be obtained by you and provided to any physician from which you seek care. Be sure to consider all the sources of care you have received in the past and make sure your physician has been provided as complete a picture as possible of your health situation. However, you will not need to provide your pharmacist with your complete medical record. The pharmacist should know your medication history and any allergies that you have to medications.

This drug history should contain all current and previous medications taken, any and all OTC drugs that you take, any vitamins or supplements that you are taking, and any herbal products that you currently take. The more complete information that you provide the pharmacist, the better care your pharmacy can provide to you. Even if you think that a medication is totally unrelated to your symptoms or what you are seeing the doctor for, be very complete in your description of everything that you take. Some patients do not view OTC medications as real drugs, but these drugs can interact with other OTC medications and possibly other prescription medications. Also remember to tell your pharmacist about any social drugs that you are currently consuming. Social drugs include the following:

- Coffee
- Tea
- Nicotine: cigarettes, pipes, cigars, and chewing tobacco, snuff, or dip
- Alcohol: beer, hard liquor, or wine

These social drugs can interfere significantly with prescription or OTC products that you might be taking. Do not hesitate to let your doctor know how many and how much of these social drugs you regularly consume. Many drugs should not be taken at all with any amount of alcohol.

## OTHER DOCTORS SEEN

Any and all physicians who treat you should be informed of other physicians, dentists, or podiatrists that you see for care. These records may be from a general practitioner, pediatrician, internist, or other specialist. The records of your care from these varying providers should be shared as needed with other physicians providing care to you. If you are moving, you can ask for copies of your medical records from your current physician and provide them to your new physician(s) when you get settled at your new location. These complete records can enable your new care providers to help you out in the optimum manner when you need care.

## OTHER PHARMACIES USED

If you happen to frequent numerous pharmacies, let your pharmacist know about medications that you obtain from other sources. For instance, if you happen to receive some maintenance medications (e.g., those for chronic conditions) from a mail-order pharmacy and medications for acute conditions (e.g., antibiotics, pain medications, respiratory medications) from local sources, make sure that all your pharmacists know the other pharmacies that you use for care and the drugs you obtain from these sources. If you obtain some drugs from Canadian pharmacies or elsewhere, let your pharmacist know about these medications as well.

## DRUGS TAKEN

Three categories of drugs are used in the United States: OTC, prescription, and herbal products.

### Over the Counter

OTC products in the United States have been approved by the U.S. FDA for sale without a prescription. These are products deemed safe for self-medication by consumers. In some cases these are drugs that previously were available only by prescription (e.g., naproxen, ibuprofen, diphenhydramine, chlorpheniramine, loratidine, hydrocortisone, etc.).

Thousands of OTCs and combinations are available for use. These products can be sold anywhere, such as:

- Pharmacies
- Food markets
- Discount stores
- Supercenters
- Small grocery counters
- Airports
- Convenience centers
- Gas stations

Please keep in mind that these medications are drugs, and they can have potent effects—both positive and negative. Just because these products are available without a doctor's order does not mean that they are not to be taken seriously and carefully within dosage recommendations—please use caution when you take them. The various vitamins and supplements available in the United States are OTC for the most part. Some exceptions include the products that contain higher doses of certain vitamins (e.g., folic acid 1 mg). Multivitamins (e.g., those products that contain combinations of numerous vitamins and mineral supplements) are widely marketed and consumed in the United States. Examples of OTC products are listed in Exhibit 4.1.

### *Prescription*

Prescription medications can be dispensed by a pharmacist only after they have been prescribed by a physician, dentist, or podiatrist. Dentists and podiatrists can prescribe only those therapies that relate to oral (in the case of the former) or foot (in the case of the latter) health or conditions. Strict federal and state rules and regulations must be complied with for the legal dispensing of prescription medications to occur. Prescription medications are often referred to as "legend" drugs. This is because they must have the following or a similar phrase prominently displayed on the container from the manufacturer of the product: "Caution: Federal Law Prohibits Dispensing without Prescription" [21 U.S.C. 353(b) and 21 CFR 201.100(b)(1)]. At a minimum, the label must state "℞ only." This requirement has been in place in the United States since the 1950s. The legend must also be placed on the prescription label that is attached to your prescription container or unit.

Approximately 3 billion prescriptions are dispensed in the United States per year. This figure excludes prescription items used by millions of patients in hospitals every day. The number of prescriptions (outpatient) dispensed each year is expected to exceed 5 billion per year in the next few years. There has been an explosion in the number of pharmacy outlets in the United States, and this trend is not expected to slow in either the near or long-term future. Future drivers of this rapid expansion will include the eventual rollout of the prescription drug coverage available to seniors through Medicare coverage for outpatient prescription medications—the Medicare Drug Dis-

## EXHIBIT 4.1. Common OTC products.

I. Acid suppression agents, proton pump inhibitors (PPIs), e.g., omeprazole

II. Acetaminophen, in various dosage forms and amounts:
   A. Oral dosage forms:
      1. Tablets—chewable and for swallowing
      2. Capsules
      3. Liquids[a]—drops and elixirs
   B. Rectal suppositories
   C. Dosage amounts:
      1. 325 mg = regular strength
      2. 500 mg = extra strength

III. Aspirin,[b] in various dosage forms and amounts:
   A. Oral formulations
   B. Rectal suppositories
   C. Dosage amounts:
      1. 81 mg = cardiac dose
      2. 325 mg = five-grain tablet (common size)
      3. 500 mg = extra strength

IV. Antacids:
   A. Aluminum and/or magnesium sulfate
   B. Calcium carbonate

V. Antihistamines:
   A. Sedating, e.g., diphenhydramine
   B. Nonsedating, e.g., loratidine

VI. Cough and cold preparations:
   A. Expectorant, e.g., guaifenesin
   B. Suppressant, e.g., dextromethorphan (DM)
   C. Containing both a cough suppressant and expectorant

VII. Drugs for motion sickness:
   A. Meclizine
   B. Dimenhydrate

VIII. Externally applied products, such as various ointments and creams:
   A. Hydrocortisone
   B. Diphenhydramine

IX. $H_2$ antagonists:
   A. Famotidine
   B. Cimetidine
   C. Ranitidine

X. Laxatives:
   A. Cascara sagrada
   B. Milk of magnesia

XI. Nasal decongestants:
   A. Pseudoephedrine

XII. Nasal sprays:
   A. Normal saline
   B. Oxymetazoline hydrochloride
   C. Phenylephrine hydrochloride

*(continued)*

*(continued)*

XIII. Nonsteroidal anti-inflammatory drugs:
    A. Ibuprofen
    B. Ketoprofen
    C. Naproxen sodium
XIV. Throat lozenges:
    A. Products that contain benzocaine
    B. Products that contain dyclonine
XV. Topical formulations:
    A. Vitamin A and D ointment[c]
    B. Vitamin E
XVI. Vitamin and mineral supplements:
    A. Niacin (sometimes referred to as Vitamin $B_5$)
    B. Pantothenic acid
    C. Vitamin A
    D. Vitamin B:
        1. Thiamin ($B_1$)
        2. Riboflavin ($B_2$)
        3. Pyridoxine ($B_6$)
        4. Cyanocobolamine ($B_{12}$)
    E. Vitamin C (ascorbic acid)
    F. Vitamin E
    G. Vitamin D
XVII. Minerals:
    A. Zinc
    B. Iron
    C. Magnesium
    D. Calcium
    E. Potassium
XVIII. Injections:
    A. Insulin[d]

[a] Never use the droppers or measuring spoons that come with these products to measure other products. Use the dropper only with drops, and use the measuring spoon only with the elixir formulations. Serious overdoses can occur if the measuring spoon is used to deliver drops of this medication.

[b] Aspirin is the most common "hidden ingredient" in OTCs. Many products contain aspirin, and it is difficult to know which ones do unless you read the labels closely or have previous experience with the product.

[c] Some vitamin A and D ointments *do not* contain vitamin A or vitamin D. Be sure to examine the section on contents to see if, in fact, the product does contain vitamin A or D.

[d] Insulin is available as an OTC product, but it is sold only through pharmacies. It must be refrigerated while in the pharmacy's inventory.

count Card (http://www.medicare.gov/MedicareReform/). An initial and modified drug benefit was provided to seniors through Medicare in 2004, and the full provision will become effective in 2006. This drug benefit for outpatient prescriptions for Medicare-eligible seniors will drive this expansion even more.

Other factors driving this significant increase in prescription-drug utilization include the following:

- An increase in the number of patients—of all ages, but especially the elderly.
- The aging of our society—we are growing older and consequently in need of more drugs.
- The availability of pharmacy services anywhere in the United States—either in person or through mail-order options and from easily accessible pharmacies in every corner of the United States.

The average rate of compliance for medications across all therapies and all age groups is 50 percent on average. Consider the increase in prescription drug use if patients were on average more compliant by 1 to 50 percent! The number of prescriptions dispensed would no doubt skyrocket.

### Herbal Products

Herbal supplements are a fast-growing consumer product line. They are available in many outlets and are popular aids to health and wellness. As with any medication or drug product consumed, you should be aware of the positive and potentially negative aspects of herbal supplement use. I encourage you to read as much as you can about herbs and herbal supplements if you use them. A good source of information on the Internet can be found at <http://www.uiowa. edu/~idis/herbalinks>. This Web site from the University of Iowa Drug Information Center is an excellent reference and informative source.

Products marketed as herbal or dietary supplements include a wide range of products:

- Amino acids
- Animal extracts
- Bioflavanoids
- Botanicals
- Nutrients
- Various enzymes
- Vitamins or minerals

Herbal ingredients of dietary supplements may include whole or processed plant components:

- Bark
- Extracts
- Essential oils
- Leaves
- Flowers
- Fruits
- Stems

These segments may be incorporated into capsules, elixirs, powders, tablets, and/or water infusions (teas). It is common to combine these products with other supplements, such as vitamins, minerals, amino acids, and nonnutrient ingredients. Unfortunately, these products may be without positive effects. They are not regulated in the same fashion as other OTC and prescription products, and are not screened for safety prior to market entry. The U.S. FDA has urged caution when using these products.

Adverse effects have been associated with these products; unfortunately a uniform mechanism does not exist to report such reactions at a national level. If such a mechanism was in place, consumers could benefit collectively from the experiences of others. Listed here are several adverse reactions that have been reported with the use of nutritional supplements. These reports have been gathered from various sources by the U.S. FDA.[1]

*Chaparral* (Larrea tridentata)

Commonly named the creosote bush, chaparral is a desert shrub with a long history of use as a traditional medicine by Native Americans. Chaparral is marketed as a tea, as well as in tablet, capsule, and concentrated extract form, and has been promoted as a natural antioxidant "blood purifier," cancer cure, and acne treatment. Numerous cases of acute nonviral hepatitis have been associated with the supplement's use. Most cases have been self-limiting; however, there has been one reported case of terminal liver failure requiring transplantation.[2]

## *Comfrey* (Symphytum officinale, S. asperum, S. × uplandicum)

Preparations of comfrey are widely available in the United States in various forms. Numerous cases of hepatic blood obstruction associated with comfrey use have occurred over the past two decades.[3] Several countries (the United Kingdom, Australia, Canada, and Germany) have recently restricted the sale of comfrey.

## *Yohimbe* (Pausinystalia yohimbe)

Yohimbe is a tree bark containing a variety of pharmacologically active chemicals that is marketed as a male potency enhancer. Serious adverse effects, including renal failure, seizures, and death have been reported to the FDA regarding products containing yohimbe. These are currently under investigation.[4]

At high doses, yohimbine (the active ingredient in yohimbe) is what is termed a monoamine oxidase inhibitor (MAOI). MAOIs cause serious reactions when taken with red wine, cheese, and/or beer. The reaction also occurs with the combination of yohimbine and pseudoephedrine (a common nasal decongestant). The reaction leads to a hypertensive crisis.

## *Ginkgo* (Ginkgo biloba)

Ginkgo has been marketed as an agent to help relieve tension and anxiety, improve mental alertness, elevate mood, and restore energy. Some possible side effects are headache, dizziness, heart palpitations, GI disturbances, and dermatologic reactions. Ginkgo biloba is considered a 2 million-year-old living fossil; it has not changed in that period of time. It was first used medicinally centuries ago in the Orient; it was used in Western medicine after its "discovery" in 1691 in Nagasaki, Japan, by Engelbert Kaempfer (1651-1716), a German botanist who worked for the Dutch East India Company in the 1680s. The drug was first extracted in the United States in Philadelphia in 1784, a century later. Kaempfer first used the word ginkgo after he was in Japan. He transported seeds to Europe, and a ginkgo tree planted in 1730 exists to this day in the University of Utrecht Botanical Garden.

## *Lobelia* (Lobelia inflata)

Lobelia, also known as Indian tobacco, contains pyridine-derived alkaloids, primarily lobeline. Lobeline exerts roughly 25 percent of the activity of nicotine, also a substance obtained from lobelia species. A "cousin" of nicotine, lobeline should not be consumed by children, pregnant females, or individuals with cardiac problems.

## *Willow Bark*

Willow bark has long been used for pain relief, fever reduction, and anti-inflammatory properties. If this sounds similar to what you know about aspirin (acetylsalicylic acid), that is because it shares similar properties with aspirin. Although aspirin is now synthetically produced, the manufactured product shares properties with willow bark. Unfortunately, willow bark is promoted as an aspirin-free supplement, thus deceiving those who use it. This substance should not be used in children or aspirin-sensitive or aspirin-allergic adults. Willow bark contains salicin, which converts chemically to salicylic acid after it is consumed. All salicylates are chemically related to aspirin. Aspirin-sensitive individuals can develop life-threatening reactions     . (such as bronchospasms) when consuming aspirin or aspirin-related compounds.

## *Ma Huang* (Ephedra sinica)

Ma huang is one of several names for herbal products containing members of the genus *Ephedra*. These evergreen plants are called by many names, including squaw tea and Mormon tea. Serious adverse effects, including hypertension (elevated blood pressure), palpitation (rapid heart rate), neuropathy (nerve damage), myopathy (muscle injury), psychosis, stroke, and memory loss, have been reported to the FDA regarding products containing ma huang as an ingredient. These reports are currently under investigation.[5] Ephedra-containing supplements were promoted as a weight-loss aid. Several deaths in prominent athletes caused a much-needed response to the sale of ephedra-containing products. In 2003, these products were banned from sale in the United States.

## Vitamins and Minerals

Safe levels of vitamin and mineral dietary supplements are established through what are termed recommended daily allowance (RDA) values. The range between safe to toxic levels can be small for some supplements.

*Vitamin A.* Vitamin A is found in several forms in dietary supplements. Adverse effects associated with taking more than recommended (>25,000 international units [IUs]) include

- birth defects in infants whose mothers consumed vitamin A during pregnancy,
- bone and cartilage damage,
- elevated intracranial pressure, and
- severe liver injury (including cirrhosis).

Children and pregnant women are especially vulnerable to vitamin A overdosing. Pregnant women should not exceed 8,000 IUs.

*Vitamin $B_6$.* Neurologic toxicity has been reported in vitamin B overdose situations; symptoms may include balance disturbances and nerve damage. The RDA for Vitamin $B_6$ is 2 mg; some formulations contain 250-500 mg.

*Niacin (nicotinic acid and nicotinamide).* Niacin taken in high doses is known to cause

- gastrointestinal distress: burning pain, cramping, diarrhea, nausea, vomiting, bloating
- mild to severe liver damage
- intense facial flushing

*Selenium.* Selenium in high doses (approximately 800 to 1,000 micrograms daily) can cause tissue damage, especially in tissues or organs that concentrate the element.

*Iron.* Iron supplements (ferrous gluconate, ferrous sulfate) have caused symptoms associated with hemosiderosis, such as coughing up blood, persistent cough, runny nose, and/or chronic fatigue. Hemochromatosis (iron overload, bronze diabetes) is a rare but potentially fatal condition whereby iron levels reach toxic levels in individuals who cannot eliminate the elemental iron. Symptoms may include increased facial hair (men or women), skin discoloration, and/or hepatomegaly (enlarged liver). The deposition of iron in lung tissue leads to rapid and extremely painful death in severe cases. The hepatomegaly will resemble alcoholic cirrhosis of the liver, even in teetotalers. Treatment of hemochromatosis involves painful and lengthy recurrent phlebotomy treatments. This is not unlike frequent blood donations, only the blood drawn is of no use to other patients. The individual is continually monitored for safe levels of hemoglobin, and also for hematocrit values. There is no cure for this condition, only supportive treatment and frequent phlebotomies.

## OTHER CONSIDERATIONS

### When Your Medication Looks Different

Depending on the prescription medications that you take, the manufacturer may change its appearance from time to time. If this happens, your pharmacist should always alert you to the change. A brand-name prescription medication (e.g., Lipitor) is rarely altered in color, shape, or size. It can happen by the manufacturer's choice, but it is extremely rare. Sometimes products are reformulated and thus require a change in the product. Most of the time, however, products are almost always the same in appearance from one time to another.

A generic medication often may be a different color, shape, or size from one refill to another. Your pharmacist may use another generic drug manufacturer, the generic drug supplier may obtain a different company's product (it is the same active ingredient, the supplier may be different), or a manufacturer may stop offering a generic product—thus requiring the pharmacist to obtain a different manufacturer's product.

If you notice a difference in the appearance of your medication from one refill to the next, ask your pharmacist about it if you have not been told about the difference. A mistake may have been made by the pharmacist in the filling of your prescription. Always examine the medications that you are prescribed for differences in appearance from your previous experience with the drug whether you are obtaining a prescription for a tablet, capsule, ointment, liquid, or some other form of a drug product. If the pharmacist cannot or will not tell you why there is a difference, he or she may be trying to hide something

**KEY POINT**

*Your prescription medications should appear the same from one refill to the next; if it differs ask your pharmacist for the reason.*

or may not want to admit that a mistake was made in the filling of your prescription. Ask to speak to the pharmacist in charge.

### What Things Are My Physician and Pharmacist Not Likely to Tell Me About Medications?

Every drug product available has the potential to work in the fashion as it has been approved, work better than planned, have a diminished effect, not work at all, or in fact have an action that is detrimental to your health. No one can predict with 100 percent certainty what the response will be when you take the medication. Your physician or pharmacist will rarely inform you that a drug most likely will not work for you, or worse yet, cause you harm. They will also be reluctant to let you know that they simply do not know enough about the drug that is being prescribed to tell you one way or the other.

It is a good practice always to let patients know the opportunities for success of the medications prescribed for them. Many drugs will have a predictable level of success associated with their administration. In other cases, it will not be possible to offer information about how successful a drug might be. I am amazed, and yes disappointed, that some physicians and pharmacists will not be totally honest with their patients about the potential for success with some of the drugs patients take. In the vast majority of cases, your health providers will openly let you know the potential for success of therapies used, and thus let you help in making the decision to use or not use a specific therapy.

### How to Obtain the Most Information Possible from Health Providers

You need to be your own best advocate when it comes to receiving health care services. Demand that you be told as much information as you need to be an informed consumer. You need to ask the following:

1. What am I being treated for?
2. What is the prescribed drug supposed to do for me?
3. Will it interfere with other drugs that I take?
4. How long will I have to take it?
5. When can I expect to see results from taking the medication?
6. What side effects, if any, can I expect with this drug?
7. What are the chances of this drug's success in treating my condition?
8. Should I take this drug with food, or are there other considerations?
9. Is a generic equivalent available for this drug that can save me money and be equally effective?
10. How can I take this drug to achieve optimal compliance and effectiveness?

These are ten simple questions for which you deserve the greatest amount of information possible. You may need to ask the pharmacist for the answers to some of these questions; regardless, it is important that you know the answers to each of them. It may not be possible to obtain a satisfactory answer that meets your specific needs through conversations with only your pharmacist or physician. By being your own best health advocate, you can fill in the blanks through your own reading, research on the Internet, or elsewhere.

Do not be afraid of letting your health professionals know what you know and where you found the information. At the same time, be open to advice and information that they provide to you. Be aware that not all the information in print or on the Internet is reliable. When in doubt, double-check your resources to find out as much as you can from other informative sources.

If you are unable to consume certain drugs due to religious beliefs, let your caregivers know about your wishes concerning these substances in advance of receiving prescriptions. For example, you may not be able to consume any alcohol; if this is the case, your pharmacist may be able to make liquid preparations without any alcoholic excipients (ingredients). Alcohol-free preparations with the same active ingredient are often available. Do not hesitate to let your pharmacist know your needs, and that you expect the pharmacy to provide you with an alternative "vehicle" or carrier for your prescribed medication. If an alcohol-free option is not available, you should expect your pharmacist to contact your prescribing physician to pursue alter-natives.

### Drugs from Foreign Sources

I cannot urge you strongly enough to be very cautious about the drugs that you obtain from foreign sources. The quality of many of these substances is suspect. Recently, the U.S. FDA issued a warning about two drugs that were obtained from Mexico and found to be subpotent.[6] The FDA warned the public about counterfeit versions of the drugs Zocor (simvastatin) and carisoprodol that were imported from Mexico by individuals trying to save money. Tests indicated that the counterfeit Zocor did not contain any active ingredient and that the counterfeit carisoprodol differed in potency when compared to the authentic product. Carisoprodol is a drug used in the treatment of painful musculoskeletal conditions, and Zocor is a cholesterol-lowering drug. The counterfeit versions were reportedly purchased at Mexican border-town pharmacies and sold under the names Zocor 40/mg (lot number K9784, expiration date November 2004), and carisoprodol 350/mg (lot number 68348A). Patients who rely on these counterfeit versions of the drugs could develop serious health problems (with the counterfeit Zocor) or have insufficient pain relief (with the counterfeit carisoprodol).

The FDA has repeatedly expressed its concern about the purchase of drugs from foreign countries by Americans. As demonstrated by this incident, purchasers cannot assume that the products meet the quality, efficacy, and safety standards of FDA-authorized products or that the FDA is assuring the quality, safety, and efficacy of products purchased from outside the United States.

Medications purchased within the U.S. system for prescription drugs have undergone rigorous testing and review to verify their iden-tity, potency, and purity and to ensure that they are safe and effective for their intended use. In addition, safeguards help maintain the integ-rity of the products while in transit to pharmacies and prior to dis-pensing to patients. Further, labeling varies from country to country, and in some cases the labeling required by the U.S. FDA is more stringent than requirements elsewhere.

Anyone who has purchased the previously described versions of Zocor 40/mg and carisoprodol 350/mg from Mexican pharmacies should consult with his or her physician as well as notify the local FDA field office. The FDA is investigating this matter and working with the Mexican authorities to ensure that further sale and importation of these products is halted.

Drugs obtained from Canadian pharmacies may be just as safe as any American product. If you do purchase drugs from Canada, use reputable pharmacies, not storefront operations that are not pharmacies at all, but are simply set up to serve as a broker between consumers in the United States and Canadian sources and that may or may not be a licensed pharmacy in Canada. This is a very contentious and hotly debated situation that will not go away until prices for medications in the United States are lowered to levels customary in other countries. If the drugs are the same and are obtained from reputable, licensed Canadian pharmacies, then you should be okay. The cartoon in Figure 4.1 relays some of the frustration people feel regarding importing drugs for personal use and potential legal barriers to doing so.

Be very cautious about obtaining drugs through the Internet. Recently, the National Association of Boards of Pharmacy (NABP) set in

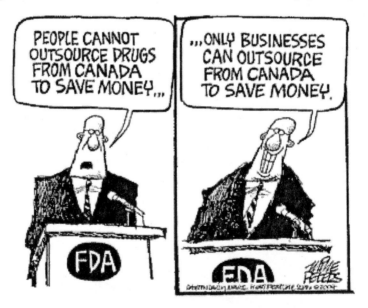

FIGURE 4.1. Cartoon highlighting the hypocrisy surrounding Canadian drug purchases. *Source:* Reprinted with special permission of King Features Syndicate.

place a process for consumers to verify the integrity of Internet pharmacies. The NABP represents all U.S. boards of pharmacy. The program, Verified Internet Pharmacy Practice Sites (VIPPS), is accessible to consumers via <http://www.nabp.net/vipps/intro.asp>. Pharmacies must submit an extensive application for consideration to be approved by the NABP. You can trust this agency to do a very good job of screening applicants, and those pharmacies receiving the VIPPS seal are appropriately licensed, have agreed to comply with federal and state laws and regulations, and have also agreed to follow the good pharmacy practices set forth by VIPPS.

---

**KEY POINT**

*Only 15 verified Internet pharmacies (VIPPS certification) are in operation at present. I would not recommend use of an Internet pharmacy for your prescription needs.*

---

NABP suggests the following are telltale signs of problems with Internet pharmacies:

- Suspect e-pharmacies will dispense prescription medications without requiring you to mail in a prescription, or they may not contact your doctor to obtain a valid prescription orally. Some send you medication based solely on an online questionnaire without you having a preexisting relationship with a doctor and the benefit of a physical examination.
- If the online pharmacy does not have a toll-free phone number as well as a street address posted on its site, keep clicking. If the only means of communication between you and the pharmacy is by e-mail, your scam bells should be ringing. NABP says that illegal pharmacy sites frequently sell their customer lists to other illegitimate online businesses, so if you buy from a sham site, you could be marking yourself as a scam target.
- If a site does not advertise the availability of pharmacists for medication consultation, it should be avoided. Legitimate sites allow consumers to contact pharmacists if they have questions about their medications.
- Be leery of online pharmacies that sell a limited number of medications. Although pharmacies may not sell every medication

available in the United States, those that specialize in medications that treat sexual dysfunction or assist in weight loss, for example, may not be operating legitimately.

In addition, the National Consumers League (NCL) Web site (www. nclnet.org) offers some tips: First, know the size, shape, color, and taste of your prescription pills. Check any differences with your doctor or pharmacist. Also, check for altered or unsealed containers, changes in packaging, or labels that appear out of the ordinary (e.g., smudged, discolored, uneven coloration, poor legibility).

The U.S. FDA Center for Drug Evaluation and Research has cautioned against buying several drugs over the Internet or from foreign sources.[7] These drugs carry special monitoring requirements or have specific safety controls on their use in the United States that may not be required elsewhere. The list includes these drugs:

- Accutane (isotretinoin), used for severe acne
- Actiq (fentanyl citrate), used for severe cancer pain
- Clozaril (clozapine), used for severe schizophrenia
- Humatrope (somatropin for injection), used for non-growth-hormone-deficient short stature
- Lotronex (alosetron hydrochloride), used for severe irritable bowel syndrome in women
- Plenaxis (abarelix for injectable suspension), used for the treatment of advanced symptoms of prostate cancer
- Thalidomid (thalidomide), used for acute treatment of moderate to severe erythema nodosum leprosum (a condition that sometimes develops in patients with leprosy)
- Tikosyn (dofetilide), used for cardiac arrhythmias
- Tracleer (bosentan), used for severe pulmonary hypertension
- Xyrem (sodium oxybate), used for cataplexy in narcoleptic patients

If you have a question about whether a drug is approved for use in the United States, you can access the U.S. FDA's current Web site (http//www.fda.gov/cder/ob/default.htm), which lists all approved drugs in the United States. If you have additional questions about the process of compiling this information, you can obtain help from the following source:

Food and Drug Administration
Freedom of Information Office, HFI-35
5600 Fishers Lane
Rockville, MD 20857
Telephone: (301) 827-6500

The FDA Web site accesses the U.S. FDA Electronic Orange Book, the compilation of "Approved Drug Products with Therapeutic Equivalence Evaluations" and the generic equivalents and manufacturers meeting FDA guidelines for marketing and sale of a drug in the United States. You can access information about both prescription and OTC products through the Web site and find out the patent status of the product. The interactive site allows you to enter either a brand name or a generic name for the drug products, and access information.

In summary, all of your caregivers need to know who else you are seeing for care, what they are providing for you, and all medications that you are taking. Remember, any substance—prescription, OTC, herbal product or supplement, and social drugs—needs to be listed for your health care providers to see. Your pharmacist especially needs to review all the medications or drugs that you are consuming and how often you take them.

# Chapter 5

# Dangerous Drug Interactions

When one drug is taken with another drug and the combination alters the actions of either drug, a drug interaction is said to occur. Any drug can interact with another drug and cause problems ranging from minor to severe—it all depends on the drug and what it is taken with. The activity of a drug can be affected by foods, beverages, OTC medications, or other prescription medications. Often physicians are not aware of these interactions. Pharmacies have computer programs that alert the pharmacist at the time the prescription is filled if interactions are possible with varying medications, but these warnings can be overridden with a few keystrokes by the pharmacist and the prescription dispensed despite the warning. Also, if a nonpharmacist is entering the data into the prescription database, he or she will not have the expertise necessary to recognize the severity of the interaction. This is another very good reason why you should choose your pharmacist carefully. Does he or she have the time to adequately examine your prescription profile (listing of all prescriptions that you are taking) and examine how a new prescription will affect the other medications that you are taking? If a pharmacist seems too busy to answer your questions about drug interactions, this is a "red flag" warning that he or she may not have adequate time to review your records.

If you use more than one pharmacy to fill your prescriptions, make sure that all your pharmacists know the drugs that you are taking, both prescription and OTC. OTC medications are rarely if ever entered into a pharmacy computer system. Since OTCs can be purchased anywhere, your pharmacist may not know which OTC medications you are taking on a regular basis. Again, OTCs are drugs and should be treated as such; let your caregiver know what you are taking and how much. By all means, if you have a question about whether a drug can be taken with another drug, ask your pharmacist.

If they do not know the answer immediately, they will surely know where to look to find the information.

## GENERAL DRUG–DRUG INTERACTIONS

Here I am referring to prescription drugs interacting with prescription drugs. Drug interactions are scaled based on severity from 1 to 5: a level 1 interaction is serious and a level 5 interaction is much less severe. As noted previously, all pharmacies that have computerized patient records have systems that evaluate these potential interactions. Many of these programs will provide the pharmacist with information on where to look for further details regarding the interaction severity. Often a medical literature source will be listed where the pharmacist can obtain more information about the drug interaction.

As a result of the pharmacist's research on the interaction between medications, you may have a small, brightly colored label attached vertically or horizontally next to the prescription label that appears on your medication container. Often these small labels will alert you to how the medication should be taken:

- For the eyes
- For oral use
- For rectal use
- For vaginal use

There may be storage or preparation cautions:

- Shake well
- Shake gently
- Keep refrigerated

Sometimes you may be cautioned:

- Don't take with aspirin
- Don't take with alcohol
- Don't take with grapefruit juice
- Don't take with antacids

Finally, instead of these text advisories, there may be a picture with a diagonal line across it, which indicates that you should not combine this prescription with the substance (see Figure 5.1). This label might appear differently, but the messages are: do not take this prescription with alcoholic beverages or do not use with tobacco products.

The use of these and other such labels is prompted to pharmacists by the computer program or, because of their education and training, they know that the labels should be applied in order to help you comply with the instructions that accompany your prescription. In some cases, you may be provided with a leaflet that lists some of the cautions that may be applicable to your prescription. If you have any questions about these labels or instructions, you can always speak with your pharmacist to clarify this information.

Two or more drugs when taken together may not affect each other at all; may have an antagonistic effect; may have an additive effect (the effects of the drug may add together to enhance each effect); or may have a synergistic effect (the drugs together have much more of an effect than simply an additive effect).

If an antagonistic effect occurs, the activity of one or both of the consumed drugs is diminished. An example of an antagonistic effect would be when a drug such as esomeprazole magnesium (Nexium) is taken with a drug such as celecoxib (Celebrex). The esomeprazole is taken to reduce the symptoms of gastroesophageal reflux disease (GERD), and celecoxib may be taken for arthritis or perhaps another type of chronic pain. The celecoxib may increase acid production in

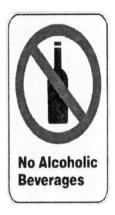

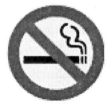

FIGURE 5.1. Examples of prescription warning labels.

the stomach, thus increasing the symptoms of GERD and negating the effect of the esomeprazole.

If the effect is synergistic, the effects of the combination may be much more intense than either effect alone. Examples may include a drug such as diphenhydramine (Benadryl), an antihistamine, and a sleep medication such as Halcion (triazolam) taken at the same time, causing increased drowsiness. Each can cause drowsiness, but the combination can make a person even more sleepy. I would not recommend that these two drugs be taken together. Nonsedating antihistamines are available, including Claritin (now available as an OTC product), Clarinex, Zyrtec, Semprex, or Allegra.

In addition, taking a sedating antihistamine with alcohol will intensify the effects of the two substances. The same holds true for alcohol taken with a drug to reduce anxiety, such as diazepam, lorazepam, or other similar drugs.

The important thing to consider with drug interactions is that a reaction could occur with your medications even though such a reaction has not been chronicled. Individuals respond to drugs individually: what affects you might not affect others and vice versa.

---

**KEY POINT**

*Any drug can interact with other drugs that you might be taking. Be sure to check with your pharmacist and physician when you have questions.*

---

## SPECIFIC DRUG–DRUG INTERACTIONS

Thousands of interactions could be listed here. Many books, summaries, and compendia have been written that specifically address drug interactions. What I will do is chronicle the most significant interactions, and again qualify that there are many, many more drugs that can and do interact.

As a general rule, drugs from the same class of drugs should not be taken together. Also, drugs that are used to treat the same ailment should not generally be taken at the same time. This is true regardless of whether they are antibiotics, drugs to treat arthritis (such as NSAIDs or COX-2 inhibitors), oral hypoglycemics, diuretics, drugs to treat depression, drugs to treat anxiety, or drugs to help you sleep.

Pain medications should also not be combined together. Pain medications and drugs to treat anxiety or depression should be used together cautiously, if at all. The effects of these combined drugs are just too intense, and it is not safe to combine them. Never take drugs from the same class together, whether they are prescription or OTC products.

Some drugs may be prescribed by your doctor in combination because they may make each drug work better (synergism) in a positive fashion. Here an example might be drugs to treat pain (narcotic analgesics or others) and a tricyclic antidepressant (TCA) drug such as amitriptyline (Elavil) or an antidepressant such as doxepin (Sinequan). Please do not combine these drugs unless your doctor has ordered them both for you.

The reactions listed here are classified as significance category 1, which is the highest-alert categorization. If after reading this listing you have a question about specific drugs you are taking, please contact your physician and pharmacist for further help and clarification. The data for this compilation have come from various sources that are listed as they are used.

### *Cisapride*

Cisapride (Propulsid) and astemizole (Hismanal) or terfenadine (Seldane) (not available in the United States, but is available in Canada and the United Kingdom). These two drugs can be obtained elsewhere, so be cautious *not to take* them with cisapride.[1] This combination can lead to life-threatening cardiac arrhythmias, including torsades de pointes.

### *Pseudoephedrine, Phenylephrine, or Isometheptene*

Pseudoephedrine (Sudafed), phenylephrine (Neo-Synephrine), or isometheptene mucate (an ingredient in Midrin) *should not* be taken with any of the members of the class of drugs known as monoamine oxidase inhibitors. MAO inhibitors include the following:

- Isocarboxazid (Marplan)
- Phenelzine (Nardil)
- Tranylcypromine (Parnate)

This combination of drugs can lead to severe headache, high blood pressure, high fever, and/or hypertensive crisis (life-threatening increase in blood pressure).

### *Methotrexate*

Methotrexate *should not* be taken with any of the members of the NSAID drug grouping.[2] The potential for toxicity with the drug methotrexate can occur with this combination. NSAIDs include any of the following:

- Diclofenac (Voltaren)
- Etodolac (Lodine)
- Fenoprofen (Nalfon)
- Ibuprofen
- Indomethacin (Indocin)
- Ketoprofen (Orudis)
- Ketorolac (Toradol)
- Meclofenamate
- Mefenamic acid (Ponstel)
- Nabumetone (Relafen)
- Naproxen (Naprosyn)
- Oxaprozin (Daypro)
- Piroxicam (Feldene)
- Sulindac (Clinoril)
- Tolmetin (Tolectin)

### *Beta Blockers (β Blockers)*

Beta blockers *should not* be taken with verapamil (Calan).[3] Beta blockers include these drugs:

- Acebutolol (Sectral)
- Atenolol (Tenormin)
- Betaxolol (Kerlone)
- Carteolol (Cartrol)
- Esmolol (Brevibloc)
- Metoprolol (Lopressor)
- Nadolol (Corgard)
- Penbutolol (Levatol)

- Pindolol (Visken)
- Propranolol (Inderal)
- Timolol (Blocarden)

The effects of both drugs may be increased. If taken together, your cardiac function should be monitored closely and the doses of both drugs perhaps decreased.

Also, beta blockers should not be taken with clonidine (Catapres).[4] Beta blockers work on beta$_2$ adrenergic receptors, and clonidine works on a$_2$ adrenergic receptors, thus the activity of the beta blockers leaves the action of clonidine "unopposed," with the potential effect of a dramatic increase in blood pressure.

### *Sertraline*

Selective serotonin reuptake inhibitors (SSRIs) such as sertraline (Zoloft) *should not* be taken with a series of drugs called sympathomimetics.[5] These agents taken with an SSRI can lead to a dramatic increase in blood pressure. Sympathomimetics include these drugs:

- Amphetamine
- Benzphetamine
- Dextroamphetamine
- Diethylproprion
- Methamphetamine
- Phendimetrazine
- Phentermine

Sertraline also *should not* be taken with MAO inhibitors.[6] (See the list of MAO inhibitors given previously.) In addition, sertraline *should not* be taken with 5-HT1 receptor agonists.[7] These agents include the following drugs:

- Almotriptan (Axert)
- Eletriptan (Relpax)
- Frovatriptan (Frova)
- Naratriptan (Amerge)
- Rizatriptan (Maxalt)
- Sumatriptan (Imitrex)
- Zolmitriptan (Zomig)

A syndrome known as "serotonin syndrome" may occur with this combination of drugs. This syndrome is characterized by central nervous system irritability, increased muscle tone, shivering, altered consciousness, and/or myoclonus (muscle jerking).

### *Trazodone*

Trazodone (Desyrel) is an antidepressant. Trazadone should not be taken with the following: carbamazepine (Tegretol), indinavir (Crixivan), ketoconazole (Nizoral), or ritonavir (Kaletra, Norvir).[8] Carbamazepine is a drug used to treat seizures or a painful condition known as trigeminal neuralgia. Ketoconazole is an antifungal agent. Indinavir and ritonavir are used to treat autoimmune deficiency syndrome (AIDS)–HIV-positive condition. If you take these drugs in combination with trazodone you may experience low blood pressure, nausea, temporary loss of consciousness (due to high blood levels of trazodone), or decreased effectiveness of trazodone (due to lowered blood levels).

### *Potassium-Sparing Diuretics*

Potassium-sparing diuretics *should not* be taken with ACE inhibitors.[9] The levels of potassium may reach dangerously high levels with this combination of drugs. Potassium-sparing diuretics (those that do not enhance the elimination of potassium through the kidneys and urine) include these drugs:

- Amiloride (Midamor)[10]
- Spironolactone (Aldactone)[11]
- Triamterene (Dyrenium)[12]

ACE inhibitors include these drugs:

- Benazepril (Lotensin)
- Captopril (Capoten)
- Enalapril (Vasotec)
- Fosinopril (Monopril)
- Lisinopril (Prinivil)
- Moexipril (Univasc)

- Perindopril (Aceon)
- Quinapril (Accupril)
- Ramipril (Altace)
- Trandolapril (Mavik)

## Thiazide Diuretics

Digitalis glycosides *should not* be taken with thiazide diuretics.[13] Digoxin (Lanoxin) is the main agent in the digitalis glycoside class in prominent use at present. Thiazide diuretics include these drugs:

- Benzydroflumethiazide (Naturetin)
- Chlorothiazide (Diuril)
- Chlorthalidone (Thalitone)
- Hydrochlorothiazide (HydroDIURIL)
- Hydroflumethiazide (Diucardin)
- Indapamide (Lozol)
- Methychlothiazide (Enduron)
- Metolazone (Zaroxolyn)
- Polythiazide (Renese)
- Trichlormethiazide (Naqua)

Cardiac glycosides taken with thiazide diuretics may effect electrolyte levels and predispose you to cardiac arrhythmias.[14]

Thiazide diuretics also *should not* be taken with cisapride (Propulsid). Here, too, cardiac arrhythmias (including torsades de pointes) may occur with this combination.

## Loop Diuretics

Loop diuretics *should not* be taken with digoxin. Here again, the diuretic effect upon electrolytes may predispose you to cardiac arrhythmias. Loop diuretics include these drugs:

- Furosemide (Lasix)
- Bumetanide (Bumex)
- Ethacrynic acid (Edecrin)

### *Anticoagulants*

Anticoagulants such as sodium warfarin (Coumadin) or anisindione (Miradon) *should not* be taken with macrolide antibiotics such as the following:

- Azithromycin (Zithromax)
- Clarithromycin (Biaxin)
- Dirithromycin (Dynabac)
- Erythromycin (various, including Ery-Sol and T-Stat)
- Troleandromycin (TAO)[15]

The anticoagulant effect of warfarin may be increased—causing bleeding episodes—if taken with these antibiotics. Hemorrhaging has occurred due to this interaction.[16] Warfarin should also not be taken with another class of antibiotics call fluoroquinolones. A listing of fluoroquinolone antibiotics is as follows:

- Ciprofloxacin (Cipro) Cipro received much attention during the anthrax scare in the United States. It was widely used for prophylaxis as well as active treatment in those exposed to the anthrax spores.
- Enoxacin (Penetrex)
- Gatifloxacin (Tequin)
- Gemifloxacin (Factive)
- Levofloxacin (Levaquin)
- Lomefloxacin (Maxaquin)
- Moxifloxacin (Avelox)
- Norfloxacin (Noroxin)
- Ofloxacin (Floxin)
- Trovafloxacin/alatrofloxacin (Trovan)

The combination of any of these fluoroquinolones and warfarin can increase the activity of warfarin, which may result in bleeding episodes.[17] There have also been reports of tendonitis with the use of fluoroquinolone antibiotics when used alone or with other drugs. If you are prescribed one of these antibiotics and experience tendon pain (usually in the Achilles tendon) stop the drug and speak with your doctor before resuming therapy.

## *Pimozide*

Pimozide (Orap) should not be taken with macrolide antibiotics (please see previous listing). Pimozide is a drug taken to treat symptoms of schizophrenia. Increased pimozide concentrations leading to adverse cardiac events may occur with this combination.[18]

## *HMG-CoA Reductase Inhibitors*

HMG-CoA reductase inhibitors *should not* be taken with macrolide antibiotics.[19] HMG-CoA reductase inhibitors include these drugs:

- Atorvastatin (Lipitor)
- Lovastatin (Mevacor)
- Simvastatin (Zocor)

These HMG-CoA reductase inhibitors are taken to reduce high levels of cholesterol and substrates (e.g., low-density lipoprotein [LDL]). They should not be taken with nefazodone (Serzone)[20] or macrolide antibiotics because the side effect of rhabdomyolosis (breakdown of muscle) or severe myopathy (muscle pain) can be enhanced due to the fact that the levels of these lipid-lowering drugs are elevated when taken with either of these drugs.

HMG-CoA reductase inhibitors should also be used with caution with sodium warfarin or other oral anticoagulants.[21] This interaction may lead to decreased clotting. The anticoagulant effect of warfarin may be increased—causing bleeding episodes—if taken with the lipid-lowering agents.

## *Thyroid Hormones*

Thyroid hormones such as levothyroxine (Synthroid), liothyronine (e.g., Cytomel), liotrix (Thyrolar), thyroid (e.g., Armour Thyroid) *should not* be taken with the anticoagulants mentioned previously (sodium warfarin or anisindione). The anticoagulant effect of warfarin may be increased—causing bleeding episodes—if taken with thyroid hormones. Hemorrhaging has occurred due to this interaction.[22] A solution to this interaction would be to have your doctor decrease the dose of the anticoagulant that you are taking.

## Bosentan

Bosentan (Tracleer) *should not* be taken with glyburide (Dia-Beta).[23] Bosentan is a drug taken for pulmonary arterial hypertension (PAH). Glyburide is taken to treat adult onset diabetes. Serious liver injury could occur with this combination. Another oral hypoglycemic agent should be used in place of the glyburide.

## Insulin

Insulin, although not a drug requiring a prescription, is always ordered by a physician due to the dosing levels that must be administered for treatment of diabetes. Insulin should not be used along with ingestion of alcohol,[24] because an enhanced level of activity of the insulin occurs. This makes the sugar-lowering effect of diabetes more pronounced (hypoglycemia—low blood sugar). If you consume alcohol, it might be best to check with your physician. Drinking alcohol in smaller amounts or with a meal or snack might be an option that your physician would approve.

### Impotence Therapy Drugs

Drugs used to treat erectile dysfunction (male impotence) include the following class of drugs called phosphodiasterase inhibitors:

- Sildenafil (Viagra)
- Tadalafil (Cialis)
- Vardenafil (Levitra)

These drugs *should never* be taken with a class of drugs called nitrates, used to treat heart ailments. Nitrates include the following:

- Amyl nitrite
- Isosorbide dinitrate (Isordil)
- Isosorbide mononitrate (ISMO)
- Nitroglycerin (Nitroglyn)
- Nitroglycerin ointment (Nitro-Bid)

Fatal heart attacks have occurred when the combination of nitrates and phosphodiesterase inhibitors has been taken.

## *Oral Contraceptives*

Oral contraceptives (OCs), or birth-control pills, need to achieve a certain and continuous blood level in order to be effective. It has been found that OCs should be used with caution with certain antibiotics (e.g., penicillins) due the fact that the efficacy of the OCs might be reduced.[25] The penicillin class of antiobiotics contains the following:

- Amoxicillin (Amoxil)
- Ampicillin (Polycillin)
- Bacampicillin (Spectrobid)
- Carbenicillin (Geocillin)
- Cloxacillin (Tegopen)
- Dicloxacillin (e.g., Dynapen)
- Methicillin (Staphcillin)
- Mezlocillin (Mezlin)
- Nafcillin (Unipen)
- Oxacillin (Prostaphlin)
- Penicillin G (Pfizerpen)
- Penicillin V (Beepen-VK)
- Piperacillin (Pipracil)
- Ticarcillin (Ticar)

It might be wise to use an alternate form of birth control when taking a penicillin antibiotic just to be on the safe side. Please check with your physician for options in this regard.

The same type of precaution should be exercised when taking OCs and members of the tetracycline class of antibiotics. The tetracycline class of drugs contains the following members:

- Demeclocycline (Declomycin)
- Doxycycline (Vibramycin)
- Minocycline (Minocin)
- Oxytetracycline (Terramycin)
- Tetracycline (Sumycin)

As with the penicillins, it might be wise to use an alternate form of birth control when taking a tetracycline antibiotic just to be on the safe side. Please check with your physician for options in this regard.

The class of antibiotics called the fluoroquinolones (see previous listing of fluoroquinolone antibiotics) might be good alternatives to use for OC users who need an antibiotic.

## DRUG–OTC DRUG INTERACTIONS

These effects can also be severe; examples of these interactions are prevalent and include synergistic reactions occurring between prescription and OTC medications. As an example of the effect that is synergistic, a patient may be stabilized on the drug sodium warfarin (Coumadin), which is taken for blood clots or clotting disorders. This patient may self-medicate with OTC aspirin, and the effect of the aspirin plus warfarin is greater than the effect of either drug taken alone; the patient may thus have excess bleeding due to the synergism of the effect of the combination of these two drugs being taken together. Unless the patient has specifically been counseled by either the physician or pharmacist not to take the warfarin with aspirin, the patient may inadvertently run into bleeding troubles by consuming both at the same time.[26]

A drug taken alone without trouble can also have a diminished effect due to another drug inhibiting the first drug's ability to work. Here a drug such as tetracycline taken with an antacid containing calcium, such as Tums, will have little antibiotic activity. Dairy products consumed with this antibiotic will diminish the activity of the antibiotic as well.

### NSAIDs

NSAIDs are available as prescription and OTC medications. The status, either prescription or OTC, of the individual product may be affected by the dose of the drug. Also, some NSAIDs are prescription medications only. The effect of NSAIDs (see previous listing in the prescription drug interaction section) on the cardioprotective activity of aspirin is currently hotly debated.[27] Your doctor may have suggested, or you yourself may have decided, to take a low dose of aspirin (baby aspirin—81 mg dose) to protect yourself from a potential heart attack or cardiovascular disease. Several manufacturers market low-dose aspirin products in many forms. NSAIDs are also available to treat minor ailments (e.g., headache, backache, muscle or joint pain, etc.). As noted previously, these NSAIDs may be available as prescription or OTC products. I recommend that you avoid the use of aspirin and ibuprofen or other NSAIDs taken together.

It might be best to take the low-dose aspirin several hours before the NSAIDs if the NSAID is only used occasionally. Apart from the cardioprotective concerns about this joint drug therapy is the issue of the possibility of increased gastrointestinal bleeding when NSAIDs are taken along with aspirin.[28] If you are taking these two drugs together and notice blood in your stools or black, tarry stools, this may be an indication that you have intestinal bleeding. Also, if you notice blood in vomitus if you are sick and are taking this combination of drugs, you may be experiencing upper gastrointestinal bleeding.[29]

## *Laxatives*

Sometimes two seemingly simple medications should not be taken at the same time because of severe and serious interactions possibly occurring. Two commonly used laxatives—docusate and mineral oil—interact severely and negatively. Docusate is a stool softener and mild laxative. Mineral oil is a stronger laxative that has more of a purgative effect. Mineral oil can also be included in other laxatives, so it may be a "hidden ingredient"; you really have to know it is in the product. When these two laxatives are taken together, the mineral oil may be absorbed into the blood stream, whereas when taken alone it cannot be absorbed into the blood stream. The docusate (DSS) transforms the mineral oil into small particles that can be absorbed. These small, emulsified globules can then enter the lungs from the blood stream and lead to a very serious form of pneumonia—lipoid pneumonia. So be cautious of combining drugs without asking your pharmacist first. Because these and similar products are obtained without a prescription (e.g., they are OTCs), your pharmacist will not know what you are taking, unless you ask beforehand and inform the pharmacist of all drugs you are taking.

Some laxatives are not meant to dissolve in the upper gastrointestinal (GI) tract (the stomach), but to dissolve in the intestines. The stomach itself has an acidic pH (allows foods to dissolve), while the lower GI tract has a basic pH. The pH level determines if a substance is termed acidic or basic. Drugs can be formulated so that they dissolve in the lower GI tract alone. These so-called enteric-coated products bypass the acidic environment of the upper GI and can dissolve easily in the lower GI tract. If some drugs are caustic and capable of producing stomach upset, they are coated in such a fashion as to dissolve in the intestines. Bisacodyl tablets (Dulcolax) are an example of an enteric-coated product. Bisacodyl oral tablets should not be taken with items that will make the upper stomach have a more basic pH level. So, bisacodyl tablets *should not* be taken with milk or milk products or with antacid preparations. These tablets should also never be cut in half in order to save money. Again, the medication itself is caustic to the walls of the upper GI tract.

Also, if you are experiencing stomach pain, nausea, or vomiting ask your health providers before you use or continue to use a laxative product. In addition, if you have kidney disease use *caution* when considering the use of a laxative, especially those that contain magnesium, phosphates, or potassium.

### Aspirin

Aspirin and aspirin-containing products are the largest segment of the so-called hidden ingredients alluded to previously. Aspirin is contained in many products, and you have to look closely or ask if you do not know what a product contains. For example, Alka-Seltzer, Alka-Seltzer Plus, Pepto-Bismol, Excedrin, and Pamprin Cramp Caplets all contain aspirin or a form of aspirin. This by no means is an all-inclusive listing; it is just an example of the brand-name OTC products that contain a form of aspirin.

Aspirin, ibuprofen, and acetaminophen are three of the most common drugs causing adverse drug reactions in the elderly, and they are among the top ten drugs used worldwide. Each of these drugs can be a "hidden ingredient" in many OTC products, which might include

- pain relievers,
- cough and cold preparations, and
- migraine combination products.

### Cimetidine

Cimetidine is an acid-reduction drug that should not be taken with theophyline, warfarin, or phenytoin (Dilantin). Cimetidine can interfere with the metabolism (breakdown) of these drugs and cause them to reach toxic levels in the bloodstream. You can use one of the other acid-reduction drugs instead of cimetidine. These alternatives can include Pepcid, Zantac, Prilosec, and so on.

You should also be cautious about the use of OTC antacid products if you are allergic to milk or milk products. In addition, ask your physician about using antacids if you have kidney disease. Antacids containing calcium should not be taken by someone with a history of kidney stones or urethral (urine-eliminating conduit from the kidney to the bladder is called the ureter) obstructions.

### Nicotine Replacement Products

Nicotine replacement products are used to help you stop smoking. If you are taking a medicine to treat high blood pressure, congestive heart failure, or an irregular heart beat you should speak with your doctor before using these products. If you are taking a drug such as theophylline for asthma and are able to stop smoking, congratulations! However, you may need to have the dose of your asthma medication reduced when stopping smoking. Nicotine replacement products may include the following:

- Nicorette
- NicoDerm CQ
- Nicotrol
- Habitrol
- Generic nicotine transdermal patches or gum

### Nasal Decongestants

If you are contemplating taking a drug such as pseudoephedrine (Sudafed) to help with a cold or nasal stuffiness, ask your doctor or pharmacist about using the product if you have any of the following:

- Diabetes
- Hypertension
- Cardiac disease
- Prostate disease
- Thyroid disease

## DRUG–HERBAL PRODUCT INTERACTIONS

Much of what we know about drug interactions is anecdotal. This is especially true of drug–herbal product interactions. Herbs can be drugs as well, but when the word *drug* is used here it refers to prescription medications.

### St. John's Wort (Hypericum perforatum)

St. John's Wort is a commonly used herbal product that has an adverse effect on many drugs. St. John's Wort is used by many individuals without their physicians' knowledge to treat depression.[30] It is also a product that *has not* been proven to be effective at treating depression.[31] The supplement has been shown to decrease the effectiveness of warfarin (increased potential for bleeding episodes); result in lower blood levels of amitriptyline (an antidepressant); lower blood levels of the heart-failure drug digoxin; lower blood levels of simvastatin (a cholesterol-lowering drug [Zocor]); and lower levels of cyclosporine (a drug taken to reduce the potential for rejection with organ transplants).[32] It has also been shown to cause grogginess when taken with the antidepressant drug paroxetine (Paxil).[33] It has also been shown to lead to serotonin syndrome when taken with other SSRIs[34] or with pseudoephedrine (Sudafed).[35] Lower blood levels of the antiasthmatic drug theophylline have occurred when taken with St. John's Wort.[36] The blood levels of the drug class benzodiazepines have also been shown to be decreased when taking St. John's Wort at the same time. This has the potential to lessen the effectiveness for these drugs.[37] Benzodiazepines include these drugs:

- Alprazolam (Xanax)
- Clonazepam (Klonopin)
- Diazepam (Valium)
- Midazolam (Versed)
- Triazolam (Halcion)

In addition, a photosensitivity reaction (severe reaction to sun or light exposure) has been shown[38] when St. John's Wort was taken with piroxicam (Feldene)—a prescription NSAID.

## *Alfalfa* (Medicago sativa)

Alfalfa may be taken to treat symptoms of arthritis, asthma, stomach upset, or high cholesterol. Alfalfa should not be taken with anticoagulants (sodium warfarin). Alfalfa contains Coumarin components and thus may make the activity of warfarin stronger.[39]

## *Black Cohosh* (Cimicifuga racemosa)

Black cohosh may be taken to treat symptoms such as hot flashes, dysmenorrhea, or premenstrual discomfort. The herb should not be taken with estrogens or oral contraceptives (birth-control pills) because it may reduce the response to estrogen that is contained in the oral contraceptives.[40]

## *Echinacea* (Echinacea augustifolia)

Echinacea is an herb promoted to treat the symptoms of a cold or the flu. Echinacea should not be taken with ketoconazole (Nizoral) or methotrexate, since the combination can lead to liver toxicity.[41] Echinacea should also not be taken with immunosuppressant drugs such as these:

- Azathioprine (Imuran)
- Cyclosporine (Neoral, Sandimmune)
- Tacrolimus (Prograf)

Echinacea taken with the immunosuppressant drugs may reduce their effectiveness.[42]

## *Feverfew* (Tanacetum parthenium)

Feverfew is an herb promoted to treat migraine headaches, fever, or perhaps menstrual difficulties. Feverfew should not be taken with anticoagulants (such as sodium warfarin) since it may enhance their effect and lead to bleeding.[43]

### *Garlic* (**Allium sativum**)

Garlic as an herbal product (not a spice or cooking aid) has been promoted to treat high cholesterol, high blood pressure, and other cardiac ailments. Garlic should not be taken with anticoagulants (such as sodium warfarin) because this may lead to bleeding episodes.[44]

### *Ginkgo* (**Ginkgo biloba**)

Ginkgo is an herbal product variously suggested to help symptoms of varicose veins, intermittent claudication (leg pains due to poor circulation), vertigo (dizziness), tinnitus (ringing in the ears), or SSRI-induced sexual dysfunction. Ginkgo should not be taken with anticoagulants (such as sodium warfarin), as this may lead to bleeding episodes[45] or anticonvulsants (phenytoin, carbamazepine), as this combination may lead to less effectiveness of the seizure medications and thus have the effect of increasing seizures.[46]

### *Ginseng* (**Panax quinquefolius**)

Ginseng is an herbal supplement promoted to reduce stress. Ginseng should not be used with anticoagulants (such as sodium warfarin); this may lead to bleeding episodes.[47] Ginseng should not be taken with oral hypoglycemic drugs (please see previous listing) since it may enhance the effects of the oral diabetes medications—ginseng has a potentially similar effect.[48] Ginseng should not be taken with furosemide, since it may reduce the effectiveness of the diuretic.[49] Ginseng should not be taken with digoxin, since it may lower the blood levels of digoxin.[50] Ginseng should also not be taken with MAO inhibitors (please see previous listing) since it may increase psychoactive stimulation (hallucinations).[51]

### *Kava-Kava* (**Piper methysticum**)

Kava-kava is an herbal supplement promoted to treat anxiety or sleep disorders. This supplement should not be taken with other drugs that also may cause drowsiness or have a sedative effect. Drugs that may cause drowsiness, such as alcoholic beverages or benzodiazepines (please see previous listing), which are used to treat anxiety or for help in sleep disorders (insomnia) may have a more pronounced effect when taken with kava-kava.[52] In fact, there has been one case report of a person going into a coma when taking kava-kava and alprazolam (Xanax).[53]

### *Lemon Balm* (Melissa officinalis *L.*)

Lemon balm is an herbal supplement that has been promoted to treat insomnia and anxiety. This herb should not be taken with other drugs that cause central nervous system depression (antianxiety agents, alcohol, etc.) since it can have an additive effect with these drugs.[54] Lemon balm should also not be taken with thyroid hormones (please see previous listing) because it can lessen the effectiveness of the thyroid therapy.[55]

### *Licorice* (Glycyrrhiza glabra)

Licorice has been suggested to help ulcers and as an expectorant (removing phlegm). Licorice is also a popular candy. In *any* form, licorice should not be taken with spironolactone (Aldactone, Aldactazide), a diuretic.[56] Licorice actually antagonizes the effect of the diuretic.[57] Licorice should also not be taken with digoxin, as this may cause low potassium levels (hypokalemia), thus affecting the cardiac effects of digoxin.[58] Licorice should also not be taken with MAO inhibitors (please see previous listing) since licorice contains drug products called sympathomimetic amines; the combination may lead to a serious condition termed "hypertensive crisis"—an abnormally high blood pressure.[59]

### *Passionflower* (Passiflora incarnata)

Passionflower has been promoted to treat anxiety or restlessness. It should not be taken with warfarin since a high dose of passionflower may promote anticoagulation, which may lead to bleeding episodes.[60]

## Shankapulshpi

Shankapulshpi is an ayurvedic (the knowledge of life) preparation that should not be taken with phenytoin (Dilantin) since it can reduce blood levels of phenytoin and lead to a lowering of the seizure threshold—more seizure activity may occur.[61]

## Valerian (Valeriana officinalis)

Valerian is promoted for use to treat anxiety. When valerian is taken with other CNS depressants (alcohol, opiate pain medications, barbiturates, or other depressants) there can be an additive sedative effect.[62] Barbiturates include the following:

- Amobarbital (Amytal)
- Aprobarbital (Alurate)
- Butabarbital (Butisol)
- Butalbital (Fioricet)
- Mephobarbital (Mebaral)
- Pentobarbital (Nembutal)
- Phenobarbital
- Primidone (Mysoline)
- Secobarbital (Seconal)

Opiate pain medications include the following:

- Codeine (contained in Tylenol with Codeine #3, as well as many other pain medications, cough syrups, etc.)
- Dihydrocodeine (Synalgos-DC)
- Hydrocodone (Hycodan)
- Hydromorphone (Dilaudid)
- Levorphanol (Levo-Dromoran)
- Morphine sulfate (Roxanol, MS-Contin)
- Oxycodone (OxyContin)
- Oxymorphone (Numorphan)

## Wormwood (Artemisia absinthium)

Wormwood has been promoted to treat loss of appetite or upset stomach. Wormwood should not be taken with anticonvulsant seizure medications (phenytoin, carbamazepine). Taking wormwood may lower the seizure threshold and lead to more seizures.[63] Do not stop taking your medication to treat seizures, just do not take wormwood at the same time.

### *Yohimbine Bark* (**Pausinystalia yohimbe**)

Yohimbine is promoted as an aphrodisiac to treat erectile dysfunction. The effect of yohimbine may be enhanced by the use of the antidepressant drugs in the TCA class (please see previous listing of tricyclic antidepressant medications).[64] Yohimbine taken with TCAs also increases the risk for high blood pressure. The use of these drugs together is not recommended.[65]

Herbs and botanicals are not tested to the same degree as other medications before they are marketed.[66] They are not evaluated for efficacy prior to marketing. They can be removed from the market only if the preparation can be shown to be unsafe. Therefore, caution is in order when using herbal or botanical products for medicinal use alone, and be doubly cautious when mixing herbal remedies with prescription or OTC medications.

## *SOCIAL DRUG EFFECTS ON MEDICATIONS*

Social drugs include alcohol, tobacco, caffeine, or illegal drugs. I will touch on interactions affected by alcohol and tobacco here, and discuss only their potential interactions.

### *Alcohol*

First and foremost, do not ever drink and drive. Second, do not drink, take medications, and drive. *Neither of these should be done, period!*

One of the questions pharmacists deal with daily is, "Can I take this medication with alcohol?" Another question that is frequently asked is: "How much alcohol can I drink with this medicine?" You should be cautious of the effect of alcohol on any drug that you take.

Earlier, I noted the problems with combining alcohol and insulin therapy.

As a general caution, if you are taking a drug to treat anxiety, insomnia, or pain, the addition of alcohol will more than likely have a synergistic effect. Older antihistamines (diphenhydramine—Benadryl, chlorpheniramine—Chlor-Trimeton), which have the side effect of drowsiness, will have even more of this effect if taken with alcohol. A synergistic effect will also occur when drugs such as the benzodiazepines (please see previous listing) are taken with alcohol. Drugs taken to treat insomnia should not be taken with alcohol. These rules are not absolute, but it is always better to be on the cautious side when considering the use of alcohol with other medications. If you are taking a benzodiazepine (please see previous listing of benzodiazepines), you should not drink an excessive amount of alcohol. What is an excessive amount? This depends on you, your gender, your age, your general health, and advice that you might be receiving from your physician or pharmacist.

Dimenhydrinate (Dramamine) is an OTC drug used to avoid and/or treat motion sickness. The effects of the drug will often include drowsiness, and combining the drug with alcohol will intensify the drowsiness activity. Driving or operating machinery should not be undertaken after taking dimenhydrinate alone, and certainly not when combined with alcohol. Meclizine (Bonine) is another OTC drug available to treat the symptoms of motion sickness or dizziness. It too can cause drowsiness by itself, and this effect is more pronounced when alcohol is consumed. The combination should be avoided. Here too, driving or operating dangerous equipment is out of the question.

Metronidazole (Flagyl) is an antiprotozoal, antiinfective drug. It is available by prescription only and is often used to treat the infection caused by the parasite trichomoniasis. Metronidazole *should never* be taken with alcohol. The combination produces what is termed a disulfiram-type reaction. Disulfiram (Antabuse) is a drug used to help alcoholics avoid alcohol. Alcohol in combination with disulfiram causes violent stomach upset, severe flushing, fever, chills, severe shaking, and general discomfort. Patients who participate in disulfiram therapy *knowingly* take the drug, recognizing that it is a self-administered deterrent to drinking alcohol, and that if they do drink they will have a certain and negative reaction immediately.

Other drugs that exhibit this disulfiram reaction when combined with alcohol include some cephalosporin antibiotics, the oral hypoglycemic agent (used to treat diabetes) chlorpropamide (Diabinese), and chloral hydrate. Chloral hydrate is a drug used to treat insomnia. In combination with alcohol it has been termed "knock-out drops" or a "Mickey Finn." The combination of chloral hydrate and alcohol should never be used. The cephalosporin antibiotics that cause the disulfiram-type reaction with alcohol include

- Cefamandole (Mandol)
- Cefotetan (Cefotan)
- Cefmetazole (Zefazone)

If you are taking a medication for pain relief, such as an opiate drug (please see previous listing of opioid analgesic drugs), do not consume alcohol, or if you do make sure you have checked with your physician or pharmacist first.

---

### KEY POINT

*As a general rule, do not consume alcoholic beverages with any CNS, mood-altering medications.*

---

Over-the-counter analgesics such as acetaminophen, aspirin, ibuprofen, ketoprofen, or naproxen are widely used products. They are widely available at many retail outlets. They are also heavily advertised products in print, on the radio, and on television. As was previously noted, they are also "hidden ingredients" in many products. Unless you specifically know that they are contained in a medication, you cannot assume by just looking at the package or name of product that they contain one of these analgesic medications. It is also very common in the United States for a brand-name OTC product to change ingredients, but not the name! This can be very confusing for consumers, so always try to know what is in the OTC products that you are taking, and be very cautious about OTC analgesic properties.

Be very cautious about taking any OTC analgesic product with alcoholic beverages. The labeling on OTC analgesic products now cautions the user to consume no more than three alcoholic beverages a day while taking the OTC analgesics. Please see Table 5.1 for the

TABLE 5.1. Alcohol warning sections on common OTC analgesics.

| Product | Warning Label |
| --- | --- |
| Aspirin | If you consume three or more alcoholic drinks per day, ask your doctor whether you should take aspirin or other pain relievers/fever reducers. Aspirin may cause stomach bleeding. |
| Acetaminophen | If you consume three or more alcoholic drinks every day, ask your doctor whether you should take acetaminophen or other pain relievers/fever reducers. Acetaminophen may cause liver damage. |
| Ibuprofen | If you consume three or more alcoholic drinks every day, ask your doctor whether you should take ibuprofen or other pain relievers/fever reducers. Ibuprofen may cause stomach bleeding. |
| Naproxen sodium | If you consume three or more alcoholic drinks every day, ask your doctor whether you should take naproxen sodium or other pain relievers/fever reducers. Naproxen sodium may cause stomach bleeding. |

FDA-required warning that must appear on the packaging for the OTC analgesic products available in the United States.

Many prescription products also contain analgesic drugs. Make sure that you know the ingredients in all the medications that you take and what interactions may occur when they are combined with other drugs.

### Tobacco

Tobacco may be smoked (cigars, pipes, cigarettes), snuffed, or chewed. (Smokeless tobacco extracts a tremendous toll on those who use these products.) Roughly 450,000 people die each year due to tobacco consumption, and another 50,000 die due to second-hand smoke inhaled from others smoking in the vicinity. These are well-known effects of tobacco. Less known is the negative effect it has on prescribed drug therapy. These interactions range from annoying to life-threatening.

**KEY POINT**

*One good reason, among many other good reasons, to quit smoking now is that the drugs that you take do not work as well when you smoke.*

## Tobacco Products Containing Nicotine

It may be difficult to distinguish the effect of smoking on disease states from its effect on the drugs used to treat the disease.[67] Because of these dual effects, patients must be made aware of the influence of smoking on many physiologic, therapeutic, and disease-state processes. Studies have identified many interactions between smoking and medications.[68] One type of interaction, the effect of smoking on drug metabolism, is well documented. The primary mechanism for interactions appears to be the induction of liver enzymes by compounds present in tobacco smoke. Smokers should use caution when using drugs from the following tabulation. If you smoke, higher doses of benzodiazepines (please see previous listing) may be necessary. Clozapine (Clozaril) is a drug used to treat schizophrenia, and when used by a smoker may need to be administered in a higher dose. Beta blockers (ß blockers have been listed elsewhere; please review the previous listing) do not work as well in treating blood pressure or cardiac arrythmias when used by a smoker. Insulin is not absorbed as well in smokers and it may be necessary to increase the amount of insulin used. When used by a smoker, warfarin is cleared from the system faster, plasma concentrations are decreased, and thus higher doses may be necessary. A smoker who takes a TCA (TCAs include amitriptyline [Elavil, Endep], nortriptyline [Pamelor, Aventil], and imipramine [Tofranil]) will have lower levels of these TCAs and thus the drug may not work as well.

Female smokers who take oral contraceptives (estrogen and progestin combination) run the risk of heart attack, stroke, and deep vein thrombosis. Estrogen is the interacting drug, and so postmenopausal women who take estrogen supplementation and continue to smoke run the risk as well. Smokers should not use estrogen products.

Alternate therapy may be available for some patients who cannot stop smoking. For example, an ulcer patient could take sucralfate. It does not influence acid production, but rather coats the site of ulceration with a spongy film, thus allowing the ulcerated lesion to heal. The patient's continuing to smoke, however, will delay healing. Patients who stop smoking may need to decrease their medication dosages (e.g., diabetes patients who take insulin, or patients who take theophylline).

The precise mechanisms of these interactions remain unclear. It is not known whether the effect is caused by tobacco substrates (nicotine or others) or perhaps by other by-products of smoking (polycyclic aromatic hydrocarbons). Nevertheless, it is important for patients to be aware of what is occurring and why. They may try to stop smoking if they can be convinced that it is futile to try to influence other disease states and attendant drug therapies while continuing to smoke. Despite a medication's demonstrated efficacy in nonsmokers or appropriate compliance by the smoking patient, the negative health effects of smoking and the associated lack of response to a medication can eventually overcome and negate any drug therapy.

## DRUG–NUTRIENT INTERACTIONS

Various nutrients or nutritional products have the potential to influence the drug therapy that you are taking. Many more exist than are listed here, but these are important and worth mentioning.

### Grapefruit Juice

Much has been written about the interaction of grapefruit juice and several medications.[69] The interaction is intense enough to come into play after consuming only one eight-ounce glass of grapefruit juice.[70] The interaction is more pronounced for certain medications, and less intense for others. The important thing to consider is that not all medications are adversely affected by grapefruit juice, only certain ones.

---

**KEY POINT**

*Ask your pharmacist for advice when obtaining prescriptions. Is it okay for you to take your medication with grapefruit juice?*

---

## Statin Medications

HMG-CoA reductase inhibitors ("statin" medications) have been shown to interact with grapefruit juice. The reaction involves more of the statin drug being in the system due to a reduction in the ability of enzymes to break it down and eliminate it. So, the effect of some of the statins is more intense than would otherwise be expected. For patients taking lipid-lowering medications known to interact with grapefruit juice, there are some noninteracting members of the same class of HMG-CoA reductase inhibitors. For example, the interaction with simvastatin (Zocor) and lovastatin (Mevacor) may be more pronounced than the interaction with atorvastatin (Lipitor), and less pronounced than others such as pravastatin (Pravachol) and fluvastatin (Lescol). So, the reaction with some statins is more important while others have an insignificant effect and presumably can be taken.[71] One of the first signs of trouble with statin medications is muscle pain. Muscle pain is a symptom of myopathy. This is a potentially dangerous breakdown of muscle tissue. Excess levels of statins can lead to myopathy, so here again, pay attention to your body, how you feel, and any pain that you may be experiencing. The increase in blood levels and subsequent increase in muscle pain may be due to the interaction between grapefruit juice and the statin drug that you are taking to treat high cholesterol or elevated lipid levels.

## Amiodarone

Amiodarone (Cordarone, Pacerone) blood levels are increased when taken with grapefruit juice, which may lead to irregular heart beats (arrhythmia).[72]

## Benzodiazepines

The CNS effects of the benzodiazepines (please see previous listing of benzodiazepines) may be more pronounced when taken with grapefruit juice.[73]

## ACE Inhibitors

The angiotensin converting enzyme (ACE) inhibitor class of drugs, which is used for heart failure and high blood pressure, may have a more pronounced effect when taken with grapefruit juice.[74] ACE inhibitors include the following:

- Amlodipine (Norvasc)
- Diltiazem (Cardizem)
- Felodipine (Plendil)
- Nicardipine (Cardene)
- Nifedipine (Procardia, Adalat)
- Nimodipine (Nimotop)
- Nisoldipine (Sular)
- Verapamil (Calan, Verelan)

The pronounced effects may include flushing, headache, irregular heart beat, or low blood pressure.[75]

## Carbamazepine

Carbamazepine (Tegretol) is a drug that is taken for epilepsy and a painful condition known as trigeminal neuralgia. The blood level of carbamazepine may be increased when taken with grapefruit juice and lead to toxic effects. These may include dizziness, loss of balance, drowsiness, nausea, vomiting, or shaking.[76]

Just be aware that grapefruit juice may affect your drug therapy, ask questions, and monitor your body to see if you notice changes when starting or continuing a drug therapy.

## Calcium

Calcium is contained in many products. Milk, cheese, and other dairy products are an important source of calcium. Calcium is contained in yogurt and in calcium-fortified fruit juices (e.g., orange, grapefruit). Calcium is absolutely essential for bone growth and stability. It plays a role in preventing osteoporosis (porous bone density). Osteoporosis is more likely to affect women, but certainly occurs in men as well.

Although calcium cannot reverse osteoporosis, individuals can help to prevent further bone decay with calcium supplementation. Persons with a history of kidney disease need to limit their intake of calcium. Individuals with a history of kidney stones (nephrolithiasis) should avoid excess consumption of calcium. Others suffering from gout or gouty arthritis should likewise limit their calcium consumption.

Calcium is vital for young children and adolescents; its importance cannot be overstated. However, certain medications are adversely affected by calcium. The goal in examining this series of interactions is to not stop consuming calcium, but perhaps altering when you take your medication so as not to be affected by taking the important electrolyte calcium.

---

### KEY POINT

*You can continue to take calcium while taking certain medications, it is just important not to take them at the same time.*

---

Calcium is also contained in many antacid products. These products are too numerous to mention. But, the calcium-containing antacids can include calcium carbonate, and can be lone ingredients or in combination with aluminum hydroxide and/or magnesium sulfate. There are times when you have to take an antacid, the point is that you might need to alter when you take either the antacid or the medication that may be affected by the calcium-containing antacid. Here again, your pharmacist is a great source of information on which antacids contain calcium and alternatives that you might use in order to avoid the drug interactions mentioned here. Also, be a thorough reader of the labels that are on the OTC and prescription products you purchase.

### Etidronate

Etidronate (Didronel) is used to treat osteoporosis and should not be taken within two hours of taking calcium supplements. The timing of the consumption of calcium and etidronate can be the difference between effectiveness and ineffectiveness.

*Phenytoin*

Phenytoin (Dilantin) is a drug used to help prevent seizures in persons with epilepsy. Calcium should not be taken within one to three hours of taking phenytoin. The drug may not be as effective if taken in close proximity with calcium-containing products or supplements.

*Certain Antibiotics*

Certain of the tetracycline class of antibiotics (please see previous listing of the class of tetracyclines, which includes the drug tetracycline itself) should not be taken at the same time you consume calcium-containing products or supplements. Tetracyclines (oral) and calcium supplements taken together may decrease the effectiveness of tetracycline. Some members of this class are not affected. For example doxycycline (Vibramycin, Vibratabs) can be taken along with any food or calcium supplement. If you are using tetracycline be sure that you do not take calcium within one to three hours of taking the antibiotic.

Other antibiotic classes that should not be taken at the same time as calcium include members of the fluoroquinolone class of antibiotics. Do not take ciprofloxacin (Cipro) with dairy products (such as milk or yogurt) or calcium-added juices alone. Fluoroquinolones and calcium supplements taken together may decrease the effectiveness of the fluoroquinolones.

=====

**KEY POINT**

*Always try to take as few medications as possible. When starting a new therapy, find out how long you will need to take it. Also determine whether you can stop other medications because of the new therapy. Never hesitate to ask for help with the questions and problems that you have with your medication therapies.*

=====

## MINIMIZING THE POTENTIAL FOR DRUG INTERACTIONS

You can do some specific things to help minimize your potential for drug interactions. Ideally, all who provide care for you should know all the drugs (both prescription and OTC) that you currently are taking. Also, let your caregivers know the vitamins, supplements, and herbal products that you take on a regular basis. If you consume social drugs, let your caregivers know the extent of this use too.

Try to take as few drugs as possible. This might be difficult for some, but is it worth attempting. As the number of drugs that you take decreases, the potential for serious drug interactions also decreases. Use as few pharmacies as possible so that you can have your records centrally located. When you are prescribed a new therapy, find out from your physician how long you are to take the new medication(s). Are there drugs that you can now stop taking because of the addition of a new therapy?

Periodically review the drugs that you are taking with your physician and pharmacist. Continually ask yourself: "Do I need to continue to take this medication?" When you feel better, is it because of the drugs that you are taking? Or, have you lost weight, begun an exercise regimen, or altered your diet in a positive way? If these positive changes can reduce your blood pressure, blood sugar levels, or fatigue symptoms, would it be possible to stop one or more of your medications?

Lifestyle changes can have a tremendous, positive, life-enriching effect on your health status. If you stop smoking, you may not need to take medications for allergies, asthma, or breathing difficulties. You may have fewer bouts with respiratory infections and thus may need to take fewer antibiotics that may affect other drugs that you take. Reducing your alcohol intake may allow you to take fewer medications and make you feel better than before.

Finally, realize the power that medications have. They can help save your life, but if taken with another drug they may threaten your life and your health. Know the drugs that you take, their effects alone and in combination with other medications, and always know a pharmacist from whom you can seek answers to difficult questions regarding the drugs that you take.

Chapter 6

# New Regulations That Impact
# Health Information You Receive

Just a word or two about medical records: You will have a record of care throughout the many places that you receive health care services. Thus, every time that you see a physician, are hospitalized, or fill a prescription, a record of this activity is updated at each point of care. Please keep in mind that although your health records are the physical property of the health care practitioner (or institution, pharmacy, laboratory, allied health professional) that has compiled it, the information itself belongs to you.

---

**KEY POINT**

*You have the right to view and obtain a copy of your medical record. You and only you have the final say about who else is allowed to view your records.*

---

## HEALTH INSURANCE PORTABILITY
## AND ACCOUNTABILITY ACT OF 1996

In 1996, Congress recognized the need for national patient record privacy standards by enacting a legislative act: the Health Insurance Portability and Accountability Act of 1996 (HIPAA). The law was enacted to protect private health information (PHI), as well as to provide for other matters. PHI relates to the physical or mental health of an individual, the provision of health care to an individual, or the payment for health care of an individual. It also identifies the individual or can be used to identify the individual.

The law specified provisions designed to save money for health care entities by encouraging electronic transactions, but it also required new safeguards to protect the security and confidentiality of patient health care information. As you already know if you have received any type of health care services in the past few years, you will be presented with a detailed description of these requirements, asked to sign a statement indicating that you have been provided the information, and provided a copy of the HIPAA regulations as they pertain to the specific care that you are receiving. Regarding prescription medications, you cannot access the records of other family members; however, you can pick up prescriptions for other family members (children, spouses, parents, etc.).

U.S. federal law provides you the right to

1. request that restrictions be placed on certain uses and disclosures of your health information,
2. know that you can inspect your medical records, and
3. know that you can obtain copies of your medical records.

Be assertive when it comes to the information you wish to receive about your health and health care. You should view this as more important than other records that you value and keep updated.

Your physician must allow you to view your medical records, even if you have not paid your bill.[1] Your physician may ask that you put your request in writing and perhaps even require you to have your letter notarized. When you do request information from your medical records, be as specific as possible. There may be a nominal charge for you to have copies of your records provided to you.[2] You cannot legally be charged an exorbitant amount for copies of your records or for access to your records.

If you suspect that someone is providing your health information to others, know that this should not occur without your explicit approval. If you are on some kind of mailing list that you did not specifically join that is related to the care that you are receiving, question your caregivers to find out how someone has received information about you. Protect your health information as rigorously as you protect financial or other important information.

The U.S. government defines PHI as

> individually identifiable health information, held or maintained by a covered entity or its business associates acting for the covered entity, that is transmitted or maintained in any form or me-

dium (including the individually identifiable health information of non-U.S. citizens). This includes identifiable demographic and other information relating to the past, present, or future physical or mental health or condition of an individual, or the provision or payment of health care to an individual that is created or received by a health care provider, health plan, employer, or health care clearinghouse. For purposes of the Privacy Rule, genetic information is considered to be health information.[3]

If you are receiving care in a hospital or other health care institution (e.g., long-term care facility, independent living facility), institutional review boards (IRBs) will be monitoring the care that you receive, including the drugs that are prescribed for you. If by chance you are taking an investigational drug, an IRB had to provide approval for the manufacturer or investigators to administer or provide the drug to you.

HIPAA was passed to do a number of things, including making it easier for employees to retain health coverage after leaving an employer. HIPAA regulations also provide for increased oversight of cases of health care fraud and abuse. In the 1990s, the tracking of abuse and fraud in the health care system increased dramatically due to HIPAA provisions.[4]

---

**KEY POINT**

*Guard your medical records as judiciously as you safeguard other important materials in your personal life records.*

---

## INFORMATION TECHNOLOGY AND CONFIDENTIALITY

Information technology has eclipsed our ability to properly monitor what is being transmitted and to whom. Unless safeguards are in place, this transfer of information can have not only positive but also negative consequences. Computerization of medical and pharmacy records affords providers and institutions unique ways to store voluminous amounts of health data with little or no expansive storage necessary, as was the case in the past. Important safeguards need to be in place to ensure that only those who should see your health data are the ones who do.

Organizations should develop clear-cut, explicit policies to monitor the security and confidentiality of your computerized medical records.[5] You should be able to review audit logs of accesses to your medical records. If something does not look right to you, or you feel there should not be access available for someone who appears on this audit log, make your feelings known.

---

### KEY POINT

*Make sure you know what safeguards are in place in your pharmacy for maintenance of your privacy. Are there adequate controls to prevent computer hacking of your private medication records?*

---

In April 2004, prescription records at the University of Kansas Student Health Center were possibly accessed by a computer hacker.[6] This affected thousands of student, faculty, and staff records at Kansas University. Officials still do not know who did it and how it happened. This is inexcusable in this day and time. However, such events do occur, so it is important to find out before you seek care what type of controls your health providers have for electronic records and transmission of such.

What might happen if your records are hacked? Potentially, your records could reveal credit card information, sensitive health information, or other personal information that is sensitive in nature. This is serious, and you have legal recourse should it happen. An unscrupulous pharmacist might bill your insurer for drugs that you never receive. Therefore, it is important to guard your health information very carefully, and make sure your caregivers are also careful with your information.

# Chapter 7

# Tools or Devices to Aid Compliance

It is one thing to talk about medications, their positive effects, and potential adverse effects, but it is difficult to follow through and be compliant with the drugs that you know you should take. If it is any comfort, you are not alone: compliance with medications is extremely difficult for many patients and for caregivers taking care of patients and loved ones. Fitting in specific dosing times during otherwise hectic days can be a challenge for us all. The good news is that there are numerous things you can do to help you be compliant. Even if you have struggled with taking medication in the past, look to the future as an opportunity to help you help yourself comply better with medication regimens in the years to come.

---

### KEY POINT

*The easier it is for you to be compliant, the more likely you are to be compliant and stay with taking your medications as prescribed.*

---

## FACTORS AFFECTING COMPLIANCE

Three types of factors affect compliance: organizational, educational, and behavioral.[1] Organizational factors include the way care is provided for you: How are the clinics where you seek care structured? After receiving physician care, is it easy for you to obtain prescription medications? Is it convenient for you to follow through on the care that has been recommended for you? Educational factors refer to the quality of information you receive from your caregivers and the information you gather from other sources. Behavioral factors refer to your attitude toward your disease state, your treatment, and your caregivers, all of which affect compliance.

### *Organizational Factors*

Does your pharmacy provide convenience and ease of access for you? Is it a hassle to obtain your prescriptions? Do you have to work through a maze of aisles and barriers to reach your pharmacy? You may have no trouble navigating through these areas, and in fact may enjoy this aspect of shopping. If not, you may be less inclined to bother having prescriptions filled or refilled.

If you are able to park, readily move from your automobile to the pharmacy, and get through the pharmacy to the prescription counter, you are more likely to have convenient access to the pharmacist for questions or for dispensing of your medications.

It may be very convenient for you to obtain medications from a mail-order pharmacy. This may allow you to be more compliant and access your medications readily from your home. However, if you are prescribed a medication for an acute condition, this may not be the best option for you. Medications such as antibiotics, medications for allergy symptoms, or pain-relief medications are needed by patients quickly, and waiting for arrival from the mail-order pharmacy may be counterproductive. Chronic medications may be ideal drugs to obtain from mail-order pharmacies, but if you are unsure which of your medications are for chronic conditions and which are for acute conditions, mail-order pharmacies may not be the best option for you.

---

**KEY POINT**

*Always know which of your medications is meant for chronic use and which ones are for acute or short-term use only.*

---

Just as important as the physical manner in which you receive your medications is the need to have ease of access to a pharmacist for questions. There is nothing worse than needing to ask a pharmacist a question and not being able to talk with him or her without an extensive series of recorded messages and button pushing to wade through. If you cannot access a pharmacist through your mail-order pharmacy or through your local pharmacy, consider finding another pharmacy source.

## Educational Factors

Educational aspects of care relate to the advice and counseling you receive from your pharmacist. The more you know about the health care you receive in general and, specifically, the more you know about the medications you take, the more likely you are to be compliant.[2] You can receive advice and counseling from your physician, your nurses, or your pharmacist. It is important that the verbal counseling that you receive be concise, informative, and specific to your needs as a patient.[3] If the information provided to you is personalized and individualized, you will be more inclined to realize the benefits from your drug therapy.[4]

Information may also be provided to you through a leaflet that you receive with your prescriptions. This written information is general in nature, not specific to you individually. It provides blanket information about a drug or a class of drugs and is printed off as a drug within the specific class is dispensed. These written leaflets usually contain the following segments:

- The name of the medication
- What the uses of the drug commonly are
- How you should take the medication
- Some common side effects

The lack of adequate information that patients receive concerning the drugs they take has prompted the federal government to become involved in mandating the provision of information to patients. The OBRA '90 guidelines stipulate that certain information be offered to patients, among other tenets. Some pharmacies go above and beyond the minimum requirements specified in these guidelines. Others simply follow the basic letter of the law. Make sure your pharmacy is an overachiever in this regard.

These governmental efforts are not for lack of cause; patients simply do not understand enough about the drugs they take. Efforts to institute mandated patient package inserts (PPIs) in the 1970s and 1980s were aimed at the lack of patient drug knowledge.

However, written information alone is not the answer. Individualized assessment and interventions must be aimed at particular and specific patient needs. For example, the usual side-effect information that is provided in these leaflets, although it may be useful, is often very limited. If you need further clarification, ask your pharmacist. The worth of these leaflets has been subject to much discussion and analysis. If the leaflet is all the counseling you receive about your prescriptions, the information is very inadequate. If it complements what you have been told verbally by your pharmacist or physician, the written information can be useful supplemental material.

---

### KEY POINT

*Make sure your pharmacist provides you all the counseling you need whenever you fill or refill prescriptions.*

---

The most useful type of information for patients is a combination of verbal plus written information.[5] Here the face-to-face counseling can be augmented through written materials to reinforce the information transmitted verbally. The important party in this counseling scenario is you, the patient. You must be ready to hear and read what is meant for you. If you are too busy to wait at the pharmacy to be counseled, set up a time with the pharmacist that is more convenient. This can either be in person or via the telephone. If your medications are prepared by a mail-order pharmacy, the pharmacy must provide a toll-free phone number for you to call in order to have your questions answered. This is your right, and you should expect no less than all the information you need whether in person or via the phone.

### *Behavioral Factors*

The most difficult task any of us undertakes is changing our behaviors. Over 250 factors are related to compliant behavior.[6] Of this number, some are certainly behavioral. Patient compliance is an individual, specific response that is variable and often unable to predict in differing patients and/or diseases. Your attitude makes a tremendous impact on the outcomes of drug therapies. If you feel that drugs will not work or that your physician or pharmacist is not capable of providing care to you, chances are good that you will be less than optimally compliant. By the same token, if you believe in your caregivers and their recommendations, you have a better chance of success in complying with medical therapies. Placebos, or inert drugs, can have

a powerful effect in achieving some level of success with drug therapies and outcomes. This effect is due to patient belief.

If you are satisfied with the care that you receive, you are more
likely to have positive outcomes and to be compliant with your medications. Physician communication style and patient satisfaction with
care are both positively correlated with higher rates of patient compliance.[7] The more the care can be provided in a patient-centered approach, the more likely the patient will be satisfied with the care and
the more likely he or she will be compliant with recommendations.[8]

The more knowledge you have of your disease and the drugs that
may be used to treat the ailment, the better your chances are of being
compliant. Learn as much as you can about your disease, read all that
you can find about the disease, and always ask questions to obtain
more information. Promise yourself to change your behavior and be
the best-informed patient that you can possibly be.

Just because it is difficult to change does not mean that it cannot be
done. I urge you to prepare for success by structuring how you take
your drugs so that you can be successful and achieve optimal health.

## SPECIFIC WAYS TO IMPROVE
## YOUR COMPLIANCE

The most crucial consideration to keep in mind with regard to patient compliance is that efforts to help noncompliant patients must be
individualized. What works for one patient may or may not be useful
for someone else. Individuals are just that, so impacts upon noncompliance must also be individualized.

### Calendars

You can make this calendar as simple or as complex as you wish.
The idea is to mark when you are to take a medication on a regular
calendar, date book, or other calendar with the days of the week listed
on the sheet. There are two ways that you can do this:

1. Write on the calendar when you *are to take* the medication.
2. Write on the calendar when you *have taken* the medication.

I like to write the medication on the calendar and then either cross through or circle the notation to show that I have taken it. Do what works best for you; there is no one right way to accomplish this. An example is provided in Figure 7.1. Here the patient takes one digoxin 0.125 mg tablet on a daily basis. The patient would repeat these markings as appropriate for each day of the month. You can see by looking at this calendar that the person missed two doses in the month, on February 15 and 21. Should the patient have doubled the dose on days 16 and 22 to make up for this? For this particular drug, I would say probably not. Chances are that missing two doses in a month would not be terribly bad, but aiming for as close to 100 percent as possible with this particular medication is a good idea. A rate of twenty-six out

February 2005

| Sun | Mon | Tues | Wed | Thurs | Fri | Sat |
|-----|-----|------|-----|-------|-----|-----|
| | | 1 Digoxin 8 am | 2 Digoxin 8 am | 3 Digoxin 8 am | 4 Digoxin 8 am | 5 Digoxin 8 am |
| 6 Digoxin 8 am | 7 Digoxin 8 am | 8 Digoxin 8 am | 9 Digoxin 8 am | 10 Digoxin 8 am | 11 Digoxin 8 am | 12 Digoxin 8 am |
| 13 Digoxin 8 am | 14 Digoxin 8 am | 15 Digoxin 8 am | 16 Digoxin 8 am | 17 Digoxin 8 am | 18 Digoxin 8 am | 19 Digoxin 8 am |
| 20 Digoxin 8 am | 21 Digoxin 8 am | 22 Digoxin 8 am | 23 Digoxin 8 am | 24 Digoxin 8 am | 25 Digoxin 8 am | 26 Digoxin 8 am |
| 27 Digoxin 8 am | 28 Digoxin 8 am | | | | | |

FIGURE 7.1. An example of a calendar reminder.

of twenty-eight days is good, but with this particular medication, 100 percent compliance is the ideal. Now, if the individual was monitoring his or her pulse on a daily basis and determined that on these days it was less than sixty-five beats per minute, not taking the drug that particular day would be a wise move. In that case, monitoring vital signs on their own and looking at dosing based on the values seen, would be ideal. If you can monitor your symptoms and have approval from your doctor, more power to you; if you cannot, try to work toward this as a goal in the future.

This calendar reminder alerts you to when you are to take the medication and lets you indicate whether you have taken the medication. It does not have to be typed, and you can choose the marking system that best suits your needs. If you take more than one medication, write them all down. If you are to take some medications on an as-needed basis, write down the times and quantity that you take each day.

The use of calendar packaging has been used by some manufacturers for many years. Oral contraceptive tablets have been packaged with a calendar–blister-pack design for decades. This allows the woman to see on a daily basis whether she has taken the tablet. Also, some steroid medications have been packaged this way. This allows patients to see how many tablets they are to take on a daily basis and how many they in fact have taken that day. An example of this packaging concept is the Decadron Dosepak, which contains dexamethasone tablets that should be taken on a tapered-dose basis. This is a dosage regimen that might be prescribed for a patient stung by a bee or wasp, or who has suffered an allergic reaction. Tapered means that tablets are taken on a decreasing quantity and daily dosage level for a period of time until the regimen is completed. This allows the patient to take the right number of tablets for the right period of time, and thus avoids either an underdose or overdose of the medication.

## Diaries

Using a diary approach is very similar to the calendar option, except you chronicle the drugs that you have taken on a daily basis and list how you feel that day and the reactions that you are having with the medications you take. These reactions can be either positive or negative. For example, you can list the dose of insulin or the oral hypoglycemic drug that you have either administered or consumed, and then list what your blood sugar levels are or how you have felt during the day. This journaling allows you to reflect on changes in your health. You also might track your blood pressure daily and write the dosage of the medications that you have taken that day.

If you are taking a drug to treat depression, write down the times that you have taken a drug to treat it and list your feelings for the day. How have you been able to sleep? Are you anxious for no reason? Do you feel depressed to a great extent? Chronicle your feelings and commit them to writing. Then, the next time that you see your physician, you can report on how you have been doing since you were last seen. This gives you a reference point to discern whether you are gaining or losing ground, and how you have been feeling over long periods of time. It can be overwhelming to try to summarize from memory your day-to-day feelings without some frame of reference to guide you. Finally, if you have forgotten to take a medication, you can easily write this fact down in a diary as well. The diary does not have to be a sophisticated or expensive volume; it can simply be a collection of sheets of paper that you have organized somewhere in a systematic fashion.

---

### KEY POINT

*Use whatever method of medication tracking that works best for you. Try several methods and see if one works better than the others to meet your specific needs.*

---

### Packaging

The ease of opening a container may seem inconsequential, but if you cannot open a container in order to remove and administer a dose, it becomes a major impediment to complying. This is an important issue for many seniors, as well as others who cannot open a vial without difficulty. I have seen situations in which people find one container that they can open and place all of their medications in this one container. This is not the best way to deal with the problem. Your pharmacy has an answer to this dilemma. Ask your pharmacist about options for obtaining your medications in a container that you can open. It may be that the prescription vials are too small for you to get a good grip on and thus you cannot maneuver the cap to open it. Ask your pharmacist for a larger container or one that is longer that you can grasp and hold while you open the cap.

## Non–Child-Resistant Closures

Please know that you can also request that all of your prescriptions be dispensed with non–child-resistant closures. You can request this on an item-by-item basis or you can sign a blanket form that requests that all your containers be dispensed in non–child-resistant containers. Some vials have reversible caps that can serve either as child-resistant or non–child-resistant closures. This is a solution that your pharmacist can easily provide for you. Some mail-order pharmacies also send extra caps that are not child resistant with each prescription. Request non–child-resistant closures if this is important to you for complying with your medications.

If you have young children or grandchildren in the house, you may want your containers to be child-resistant. Pharmacies are legally obligated to dispense medications in child-resistant containers unless asked by the patient to do otherwise.

You can really be in a sticky situation, figuratively and actually, if you have a prescription for a liquid medication in syrup form. The sugar content can coalesce at the ridge of the top of the bottle and form a sticky barrier that makes opening the container difficult, to say the least. I tell patients to wipe the top with a clean cloth or towel after each use, so the syrup never has the chance to build up at the top and prevent ease of access. This will work best if the cloth is damp. A paper towel or napkin is probably not the best method, since the paper will stick to the syrupy liquid and be attached as well. Here again, your pharmacist can provide you with containers that are not child-resistant for the liquid prescriptions that you have.

Inhalers, nebulizers, and specialized sprays are available in only one type of container. Thus, your pharmacist cannot provide you with alternatives for these medications. If you have trouble with accessing these medications, ask your pharmacist for help in making their access as easy as possible. They might have a tip for you to use that simplifies the opening and access. Often, it can be difficult to understand how to use these specialized containers. It is a good idea to always ask your pharmacist for tips to help you use them properly, to your health advantage.

## Divided Containers: Specialized Pill Boxes

Several companies market divided "pill" containers. These containers have seven (see Figure 7.2), fourteen, or twenty-eight separated segments where you can place a day's, two weeks', or a month's worth of medications. These divided pill boxes allow the patient to see what has been taken on a daily basis and to place the required doses in a container in an organized fashion. The containers come with various sizes for the daily segments, so that a person who takes numerous drugs daily can place them all in the container. These containers are specifically designed to keep medications dry and have closures that help to ensure the medications stay fresh. I have to stress that these types of containers are a much better option than trying to

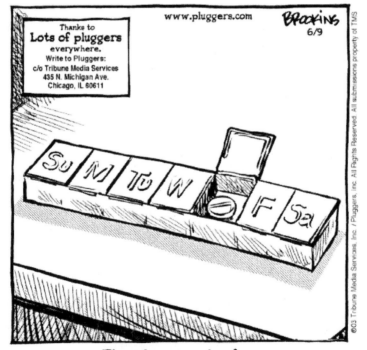

The plugger calendar.

FIGURE 7.2. Plugger cartoon. *Source:* Copyright, Tribune Media Services, Inc. All Rights Reserved. Reprinted with permission.

place medications in any type of separated container. I have seen medications placed in fishing tackle boxes. These are *not* the containers I am suggesting be used as medication separators!

One retail line of medication containers is the EZY-DOSE container products. ForgettingThePill.com also sells a complete line of these types of containers. Some containers even have timers to alert you to when you need to take your medications. Some tablets should not be placed in these type of containers, however. One such drug is nitroglycerin. Nitroglycerin tablets are taken to alleviate cardiac pain (angina pectoris). These tablets are very sensitive to light, heat, and moisture. Thus, I recommend not placing them in a separate container, even if the container is advertised as safe for any tablet or capsule. Nitroglycerin is just too susceptible to environmental changes. The stability of these tablets is just too important to risk transfer to another container.

### Electronic Monitors

Some patients are helped by memory devices. Several devices are on the market that can help remind a person to take medications on schedule. These items stimulate patients to take medications as directed. These devices vary from simple to complex. Consider using whatever works for you or the person you are caring for.

## GETTING INTO THE HABIT OF COMPLYING

A good habit to acquire is compliance nearing 100 percent perfection. You can do certain things to help yourself remember to take your medications: timing and grouping are options for you to consider.

### Timing

You brush your teeth several times a day, and the timing of this activity is similar every day. You can take your medications at the same time to help you remember to comply and to get into the habit of doing so. Taking your statin drug, a high blood pressure medication, and/or a drug to treat heart failure at the same time as you brush your teeth may help you place the taking of these drugs in a rhythm. It will be so routine for you that it becomes second nature to take your medications at this time. Are there other routine activities in your daily life that can be paired with medication taking? Pick an activity that you do daily. If you need to take medications with you to your worksite, place the medication containers in a spot that you can use as an anchor to help remind you of the next dosing interval. This might be a lunch box, a desk drawer that you access routinely, or in your purse or briefcase. By coupling normal daily activities with medication taking, you can begin to help yourself become more compliant.

### *Grouping*

It is daunting to consider drug regimens that require you to take one tablet daily, another twice a day, a third three times daily, a fourth four times daily, and perhaps yet another every four hours. If you also have a medication that is to be taken on an as-needed basis, you can see how quickly someone can become confused about what to take and when to take it! Without trying to oversimplify a very complex situation, you can do some things to help organize this. If it is possible, take all the doses for the morning regimens at the same time. You may have to take numerous medications at the same time. However, I feel that this is a better situation than trying to remember to take numerous medications at different times in the morning. Do the same grouping activity around lunchtime, supper time, and bedtime. If you are to take a medication every six hours, you can combine this medication with others that you take three or four times a day. Work at developing a method of ensuring that you remember to take the doses that you are supposed to take. Finally, if you take medications on an as-needed basis, try to take them at a similar time as you take the other medications that are routinely taken so that you can remember that you have taken it and can track the number that you take daily.

### *Count Backward to Move Forward*

If you are at a point where you simply cannot remember if you have taken all the drugs that you are supposed to take, help yourself with some facts. Usually medications are dispensed on a thirty-day basis. You might want to count the number of tablets or capsules that you have left in the container and count the number of days since you had the prescription filled. This will help you figure out how many units you should have taken and how many you have left. You can empty the container of tablets or capsules into a bowl, count them and place them back in the container. Then you can move ahead to decide if you should take the dose or not.

### Buddy System

It is also useful to have someone else help you remember to take your medications. This may be a friend, a colleague, or a family member. Have them call you on the phone, send you an e-mail message, or talk to you face to face to remind you when you are to take your medications. This technique is doubly helpful if you are taking a drug that affects your memory in a negative fashion. If your medications affect your memory, do not feel that this is some flaw in your character. Many medications have the potential to do this; recognize that it might occur, have your friends or loved ones help you remember, and always make the best of the situation.

## OTHER CONSIDERATIONS

Many other devices have been used to try to improve patient compliance. Physicians sometimes use prescriber order entry[9] with the goal of decreasing prescription processing time and increasing the opportunities for pharmacists to work with patients. Computer-generated reminder charts for patients[10] and various caps and counter devices have also been tried.

### E-Prescribing

Automatic prescription order entry, also termed e-prescribing (electronic prescribing), occurs when the physician enters your prescription information into a computer, and it is then transmitted to the pharmacy for dispensing. You need to do nothing other than simply go to the pharmacy and pick up your medications. This has the potential to decrease errors in prescribing and dispensing and make it easier for the patient to comply.

### Tablet Splitting

This has been both acclaimed and cursed as a method to increase compliance. It is acclaimed because theoretically by making your medication go twice as far, you will be more inclined to be compliant because it is less expensive for you to comply with your medications. However, the use of a tablet splitter to enable economic savings by dividing a higher-dose tablet into two smaller doses was found to discourage patients from complying because of confusion.[11] Also, many drugs are in dosage forms that should not be split. These dosage forms include capsule formulations and extended-release or controlled-release medications. The drugs in extended-release formulations are meant to be dispersed over an eight- to twelve-hour period. More will be presented regarding these types of tablets and capsules in Chapter 10. Also, some drugs are enteric-coated formulations that should not be sliced open. Drugs that are enteric coated are meant to dissolve in the less-acidic (basic) environment of the intestines rather than the stomach. These drugs are formulated this way so that you will not experience a stomach upset when taking the medication. Drugs that cause stomach upset formulated in the enteric coated form will not cause the stomach upset when dissolved in the intestine. Aspirin, some laxatives (bisacodyl—Dulcolax), and other products are enteric coated to minimize stomach upset. As an aside, if bisacodyl were not enteric coated and swallowed as is, stomach upset would be a certain outcome of the dosing. It also comes in a suppository formulation for quicker action for some who prefer this route of administration.

### Specialized Caps

The use of a notched, clicking cap for prescription medications has been shown to increase compliance.[12] These caps are a visual reminder for when you are to take your medication and a way of telling that you have taken your medication. Caps with electronic devices that can download information to a computer in order to track compliance have been used as compliance-detecting and compliance-recording tools.[13] Some of these items might be cost prohibitive for many patients and contain too much technology to be useful for many people. Other electronic devices can measure removal compliance from blister-packaged doses.[14]

## Blister Packaging

Blister packaging is a process whereby the medications that you take are heat sealed in a small compartment and placed in an accessible card, where they are easy to extract at the time of dosing. This gives you a visual reminder of what you are to take and what you have or have not taken. Blister packaging and compliance packaging have been used to enhance compliance.[15] Blister packaging and unit-of-use materials are extensively used for prescription medications elsewhere in the world.[16] Blister packs are sometimes referred to as "bingo" cards due to the similar shape and visual appearance of the medication cards.

Tablets are rarely moved from one large container to a smaller container elsewhere in the world. It is a uniquely American phenomenon. I feel it is *not* the best way to get medications to the consumer. I think because of the visual reminder aspects of unit-of-use packaging, patients have the potential to be more compliant. However, unit-of-use packaging is not without controversy; it has in fact been criticized for lack of standardization between products and manufacturers, which can confuse patients.[17]

In summary, whatever works best for you is what you should use to help. You may also combine several of these suggestions to help even more. If the calendar combined with the divided pill box works best for you, so be it. You are the final determiner of what is best for you. You might also try several of the previously mentioned suggestions to see if any works better for you with your particular needs.

For the most part, with regard to compliance-enhancing strategies—the more things that are done the better the chances are of success. Combine a memory enhancer or behavioral cue with a container aid or a calendar or diary to further help your compliance. Enhancing compliance is more art than science, and more trial and error than smooth precision. Success may be frustratingly difficult to achieve, but suitable patient compliance should be the ultimate goal of the prescribing, dispensing, and therapeutic monitoring process.

# Chapter 8

# When You Should Not Be Compliant

There are occasions when you should stop taking your medications and await further advice from your caregivers. This is intelligent noncompliance. You may be advised to stop taking the medication altogether, another medication may be prescribed for you, or you may be asked to be seen by a physician.

In other cases, because of side effects that are occurring, you may be advised to stop taking your medication and see your doctor. After consultation with your doctor, you may also be able to get better without taking a medicine.

## *INTELLIGENT NONCOMPLIANCE*

In some cases it may not be necessary for you to continue to take medications. Some drugs are prescribed on an as-needed basis. Examples here might be oral antihistamines for allergies that may come and go during the year, and thus you may not need to take the drug year-round. In another instance, the dose of a drug such as insulin to treat diabetes may require that you alter the amount injected or taken via an insulin pump.

Also, you may need to alter how you take a drug such as digoxin (Lanoxin) to treat congestive heart failure if your pulse falls below a certain minimum amount. For example, when I presented the calendar method of helping patients comply, I noted that the patient may have skipped two daily doses because his or her pulse was less than 65 beats per minute when it was self-monitored in the morning.

Other drugs such as sodium warfarin (Coumadin) may require that the dose be changed from time to time and that you be intelligently noncompliant. You may be asked to skip a dose or two; this is perfectly normal and is frequently done with many drugs. The dosing of many drugs is more art than science and may require that you be patient and try several different regimens in order to be successful in taking your drugs.

## ADVERSE DRUG EFFECTS OR SIDE EFFECTS

Virtually every drug has the potential for an adverse effect or side effect. What is the difference? An adverse effect is always a negative outcome, whereas a side effect may or may not be negative. It is important to monitor your body functions to know what effects are normal for you.

### Adverse Reactions

If you notice a change in how you feel, if you feel different, or if you notice a difference in your bodily functions, you may be experiencing an adverse drug reaction. Contact your physician and your pharmacist and explain your current symptoms and the drugs that you are taking.

This all becomes more difficult when the person experiencing a potential reaction is a young child. Obviously, children cannot always tell you about how they are feeling; you just have to try to decipher this on your own. You can see effects such as nausea and vomiting, diarrhea, or other obvious signs. Often medications may cause minor stomach upset, but be observant and look for things that may be awry. If your child appears lethargic, will not eat or drink, or is experiencing something else that is disturbing, contact your physician or pharmacist without delay.

It is a good idea to have the poison control center phone number prominently displayed at several locations where you live. These centers are staffed with knowledgeable professionals that help with any type of poisoning emergency or question—not just those related to drugs, but any substance. A very useful link listing such centers and providing further information is found at the American Association of Poison Control Centers Web site (http://www.aapcc.org/findyour.htm). Also, in an emergency you will be immediately connected to the local poison control center that is closest to where you live by dialing 1-800-222-1222. This toll-free number will work from any phone in any location to connect you immediately to the closest center.

### Predictable Reactions

Some drugs lead to a very predictable but benign side effect. For example, some drugs cause the urine, sweat, sputum, saliva, or tears to be colored (red-orange in the case of rifampin [Rifadin] and phenazopyridine [AZO Standard, URISTAT], a urinary tract analgesic taken orally) or darker in color (yellow in the case of B vitamins). These discolorations are harmless and nothing to be alarmed about. They may in fact indicate that you have been taking the medication in question.

Some coloration that might appear in your body fluid wastes is *not* normal, but rather a warning sign that something is wrong. For example, if you notice blood specks in your urine or feces, this is not normal. You should be concerned and alert your care providers.

If you are unable to urinate or defecate or are having trouble doing so (more than usual), this too is a cause for concern and you should alert your physician and pharmacist. Some drugs may have this effect on patients, but it is always a good idea to check and make sure that others know of your troubles in this regard. If you notice blood in the stool, this is cause for concern. This may be due to a mild condition (hemorrhoids) or perhaps a serious one (colon cancer). Regardless, you need to view this symptom seriously and check to find out what is causing this.

Sometimes adverse drug effects do not occur with the patient's first use of the drug. In this instance, a drug effect may have an additive influence on a patient and not occur until multiple uses of the drug, or perhaps even multiple years' use of a medication. Also, a drug by itself may not lead to an adverse drug event, but the combination of the drug plus a new medication or medications may lead to an adverse drug event.

## LACK OF THERAPEUTIC EFFECTS

Drugs that are available for use have been approved for marketing and sale by the U.S. Food and Drug Administration (http://www.fda.gov). The drugs approved are tested for safety and efficacy in human populations. However, the testing is limited to small numbers of patients, depending on the drug and condition treated. Often the sample is made up of young, healthy males. The drug is gauged to be effective when compared to a placebo or to a "gold standard" drug. A "gold standard" drug is one which is considered to be the current best drug for use in a certain disease state. Drugs are tested against the activity of the gold standard drug to determine if the drug actually has any merit over and above what is currently available. A placebo is an inert substance that is formulated to look like the same drug as the active drug in question, but in fact has no physiological effect whatsoever. It usually contains a substance called lactose (an inert carbohydrate) in either a liquid, tablet, or capsule formulation. By all appearances and even taste, the placebo is comparable to the active drug, except that it does not contain the active drug.

Drug testing against a placebo is commonplace for new drugs as they move through the approval process at the FDA. The word placebo comes from the Latin derivation: "I will please." In days gone by, a placebo or inactive substance was given to a patient to appease them or satisfy their desire to take something. Now the term is used mostly for clinical trial purposes. However, your physician may still try to use a placebo if he or she does not think that you should be taking an active drug for an illness. If you see the word placebo spelled backward on your prescription (i.e., obecalp), you can be certain that you are receiving a placebo. I personally do not favor this activity; I feel that it is disingenuous for a physician and pharmacist to use a false drug for treatment. Interestingly, the effectiveness of the placebo in many clinical trials is close to that for the active drug being tested. Simply the process of taking a drug that is prescribed by a physician, even though it contains no active substance, can in and of itself have a positive effect. It is curious just how close the effectiveness difference is between the placebo and active ingredients for many clinical trials.

When a drug that you are prescribed does not work as you or your physician expects, this is not your fault, and you should not feel that you are somehow to blame. In these cases, you may need to be placed on a different medication. Also, sometimes a drug may lose its ability to be effective over time. Great variability exists in how a drug works in general, and certainly in how it works from patient to patient. Be patient with yourself as you work with your care providers to find the best drug for you with the optimum ability to provide you with the help that you need.

## DRUG-FREE IMPROVEMENT

Also, you may find that you can feel better without taking anything or by discontinuing a certain medication. This is great; just make sure that you and your physician(s) are all on the same page when it comes to discontinuing the drugs you are taking.

Many drugs are meant to be taken for a short period of time anyway. Examples of these types of drugs include

- antibiotics, unless taken for prophylactic reasons as prescribed by your physician,*
- pain medications for acute pain, postsurgery, dental work, or similar situations,
- antianxiety medications,
- antidepressant medications (you may have to take some medications for longer periods of time),
- seasonal allergy medications, or
- drugs to treat short-term breathing conditions.

You might not need to take these or other medications for more than a few days or weeks; it just depends upon you and your symptoms.

### KNOWING WHEN YOU SHOULD
### OR SHOULD NOT COMPLY

The best advice I can give you here is to monitor your own symptoms and how you are feeling. If you feel better, are symptom free, and can alter other aspects of your life to avoid taking medications, more power to you! Think about how you felt before you started taking the medication and how you feel now. Is there a difference? Can you be sure that you do not need to take your medication any longer?

For instance, if you have adult-onset diabetes[1] and can lose unwanted pounds, increase your exercising, and alter your diet positively, you may not need to take oral hypoglycemic agents ("oral insu-

---

*Antibiotics that have been prescribed for five, seven, or fourteen days should *always* be taken until all of the doses have been used, unless an adverse reaction occurred or your physician instructed you to stop the course of antibiotics sooner than initially suggested.

lin"). If you have high blood pressure and can control your hypertension through diet, exercise, and nutrition and avoid taking pills, you will be better off.[2]

If you are taking a medication to treat depression (e.g., Paxil, Prozac, Wellbutrin, amitriptyline), do you think that you can continue to feel positively about yourself and be less depressed without the medication?[3] If your answer is an unequivocal yes, talk to your doctor about perhaps stopping the drug. There is nothing wrong with you if you feel that you still need the medication, but if you can get by without it, it might be something for you to consider doing.

---

### KEY POINT

*Do not abruptly stop any of your medications unless you are experiencing a drug interaction. If you do not think you need to continue your medication, always check with your pharmacist or physician first.*

---

Think about whether you would be better off without taking your medications. If you can answer yes, ask you doctor about alternatives. If you cannot answer yes, then you may be better off continuing on your medications and trying to be optimally compliant.

Chapter 9

# Specific Directions for Taking Your Medications

Not only is it difficult to remember to take your medications but also there are often requirements to take your medicine with food, without food, at meals, or some other instruction that may be difficult to remember. It is always good to ask your pharmacist about which medications you take are affected, or unaffected, by food intake. The pharmacist will have reference materials that can help you to decide which of your medications are best taken with food or without food.

## *TO BE TAKEN WITH FOOD*

Some medications need to be taken with food in order to be absorbed from the stomach. One such drug is nitrofurantoin (Macrodantin). Some medications have caustic effects on the stomach if taken without food, and thus your doctor may want you to take the drug with food to minimize your chances of stomach upset. Other drugs are absorbed whether or not you take them with food, so to minimize stomach upset you may want to take them with food. Medications that should be taken with food have increased rates of absorption and higher blood levels when taken with food.

Drugs that can be taken with food include the following (listing is not all inclusive; always check with your pharmacist for clarification):

- Allopurinol (Zyloprim), drug used to treat gout
- Amiodarone (Cordarone), drug used to treat arrhythmias

- Carvedilol (Coreg), a β-blocker drug to treat heart failure or high blood pressure
- Hydroxychloroquine (Plaquenil) and chloroquine, drugs used to treat malaria
- NSAIDs (please see previous listing of these drugs used to treat arthritis, muscle pain, back pain)
- Griseofulvin, a drug taken orally to treat fungal infections
- Iron supplements, taken with food to minimize stomach upset
- Dexamethasone (Decadron) and prednisone, oral steroids (corticosteroids) used for many conditions (e.g., allergic reactions to insect bites or stings, allergic reactions to some medications, severe asthma, some cancers)
- Ticlopidine hydrochloride (Ticlid), a drug taken to lessen possibilities of further strokes or temporary ischemic attacks (TIAs)
- Niacin or nicotinamide, Vitamin $B_5$, taken in higher doses to treat hypercholesterolemia or other lipid disorders
- Potassium salts, prescription-strength supplements that may include K-Tabs and Klor-Con
- Procainamide, an antiarrhythmia therapy
- Trazodone (Desyrel), a drug to treat depression
- Sulindac (Clinoril), a drug to treat arthritis
- Salsalate, an aspirin derivative taken for pain relief
- Antiepileptic drugs, drugs used to treat seizure disorders that may include carbamazepine (Tegretol), ethosuximide (Zarontin), gabapentin (Neurontin), phenytoin (Dilantin), primidone (Mysoline), and valproic acid (Depakene)

Also remember that taking with food does not mean that you have to eat a five-course meal in order to take your medications. It may be as simple as taking your medications with a soda cracker, piece of bread, or a glass of milk. It is not the quantity of food that is important, but just having something in your stomach to help the medication either work better or cause less stomach upset.

## TAKE ON AN EMPTY STOMACH

Other medications are made inactive by consumption with food; for example, tetracycline (Sumycin) is inactivated by taking it with food. Other drugs that should not be taken with food include the following (listing is not all inclusive; always check with your pharmacist for clarification):

- Penicillin antibiotics (please see previous listing of penicillins)
- Other "tetracycline" antibiotics, in addition to tetracycline itself (please see previous listing of tetracyclines)
- Felodipine (Plendil), a drug to treat cardiac arrhythmias
- Loratidine (Claritin), an antihistamine, nonsedating variety
- Sulfadiazine, a sulfonamide antibiotic
- Sulfamethoxazole combined with trimethoprim (Bactrim), an antibiotic used to treat urinary, sinus, and/or respiratory tract infections
- Loracarbef (Lorabid), ceftibuten (Cedax), cephalexin (Keflex), or other cephalosporin-type antiobiotics
- Sucralfate (Carafate), a drug to treat gastroesophageal reflux disease (GERD), or peptic ulcers
- Zafirlukast (Accolate), a drug to treat asthma

## AVOID CERTAIN FOODS OR DRINKS

Some medications such as MAO inhibitors *should not* be taken with food or food by-products that contain tyramine. Tyramine is contained in the following substances:

- Aged cheese: blue, Boursault, Roquefort, Stilton, and Swiss
- Alcoholic beverages: ales, beers (including some nonalcoholic beers), red wines (especially Chianti), port, Riesling, sauternes, sherry
- Distilled spirits (vermouth)
- Sauerkraut, yeast, and yeast extracts (marmite, brewer's yeast, and baker's yeast)

The reactions here can be deadly and lead to a hypertensive crisis (abnormally high blood pressure), as well as diarrhea, flushing, pounding chest, and/or excessive perspiration (sweating).

If you are unsure about tyramine content in foods, ask your pharmacist or doctor for information.

# UNIQUE DOSING REQUIREMENTS FOR SOME DRUGS

Several drugs are used to treat osteoporosis (bone weakening, brittle bones) in the class of drugs called biphosphonates that have specific and significant dosing requirements. Biphosphonates approved for use in osteoporosis include alendronate (Fosamax), Etidronate (Didronel), and risedronate (Actonel).

## *Alendronate, Etidronate, and Risedronate*

Take alendronate (Fosamax) or risedronate (Actonel) with six to eight ounces of water (full glass) on an empty stomach. Alendronate or risedronate should be taken early in the morning at least thirty minutes *before* any food, beverage (coffee, juice, milk), or your other medicines. Drinks such as coffee, tea, mineral water, or juice will lower the amount of the drug absorbed by your body. Also, avoid any calcium-containing products (antacids, laxatives, vitamins, milk, milk-based formulas, or any cheese products) within two hours of dosing with etidronate. These products will also decrease the absorption of alendronate or risedronate. You can continue to take these, just not within two hours of the dosing.

You should not lie down for one-half hour after taking either of these drugs. This will help the medication reach your stomach faster. It will also help you avoid irritation of your esophagus. You can sit upright; just do not lie down.

# WHAT TO DO IF YOU FORGET A DOSE

The normal inclination when you forget a dose is to go ahead and take it right away. This is not always the best course of action. Let me go through some specific examples of when and when *not* to take the forgotten dose.

## *Once-a-Day Drugs*

If you take a drug once daily in the morning, forget the dose, and remember you forgot it early in the afternoon or evening, go ahead and take the medication the same day, then resume the normal dosing time the next day. If it is almost time to take your next dose, do not double up. If you forget about the dosing until the next day, do not double up on the dose when you take the dose the next day. There are exceptions, and it is always best to check with your physician to make sure you do what you should with skipped doses. If the drug is an oral contraceptive (birth-control pill), you can ask your physician to make sure, but usually taking two the next day will suffice.

### *Twice-a-Day (or more) Drugs*

If you take a medication twice daily and you forget to take a dose, you can go ahead and take it if it is fairly close to the time you missed, spacing the dose as far as you can from the next dose administration. Do not arbitrarily double or triple the dose if you forget several doses and do not remember when you took the last dose. In this case, ask your physician for advice. If you are taking an antibiotic and you forget to take a dose, take it as soon as you can remember to do so and resume the normal schedule.

Do whatever you can to take your medications as prescribed. If you have been told specific ways to take your drugs, always ask for tips and advice that can be helpful to you in complying. Most of us take more than one medication: more than 60 percent of office visits to physicians result in one or more prescriptions being written.[1] This makes our task complicated; if we are to take medications in a special manner, this can hinder our best efforts to be compliant. That is why advice can be helpful from your physician, pharmacist, family members, friends, or acquaintances.

# Chapter 10

# Other Considerations
# When Taking Medications

Various medications may require special handling, storage, or administration techniques. This chapter presents some issues to consider with certain dosage forms that may require you to do different things regarding their use.

## *REFRIGERATION*

Some medications require refrigeration before and during their use. Some drugs for injection supplied in a multiuse container are meant to be refrigerated. Other medications may be stored in a refrigerator, but it is not necessary to do so. An example here is insulin for injection. Insulin bottles are stored in a refrigerated environment to protect their shelf life (or freshness period). However, insulin in these containers need not be refrigerated after opening, just stored at room temperature. Most people continue to refrigerate their insulin bottles, but it is not necessary. If you are traveling, you should keep the insulin in an environment where the bottle(s) will not become excessively heated. You can also purchase insulin on trips in pharmacies as you go along. You do not necessarily need to stock up in advance and try to arrange refrigeration for the insulin.

Your other medications (tablets, capsules) need not be refrigerated. Some people feel that keeping their medications in the refrigerator will assure that they stay fresh. This is not the case; in fact, the moisture and humidity present in the refrigerator actually may not be good for the medications. The moisture will affect the stability of many tablets and capsules. In fact, all prescription medications coming from the manufacturer contain sodium silicate contained in either a semiporous packet or small canister which absorbs excess moisture in the container. This is again in recognition of the need to have tablets and capsules stored in a moisture-free environment. These sodium silicate packets are harmful if swallowed, so please do not ingest them or keep them within reach of a child or a pet.

Prescriptions for antibiotics for children in liquid form are put into solution (reconstituted) by the pharmacist prior to dispensing. These antibiotic suspensions *must* be refrigerated. Other liquid preparations such as cough syrups and pain relief liquids *do not* need to be refrigerated. Some antibiotic prescriptions (e.g., sulfamethoxazole/trimethoprim) (Bactrim) also *do not* need to be refrigerated.

---

### KEY POINT

*It is a good idea to always check with your pharmacist if you have any uncertainty whatsoever about refrigeration needs for any prescription product.*

---

## STORAGE

If you are like most Americans, you had or have a medicine cabinet in your bathroom. These might be nice storage devices for some things, but not for your medicines! The cabinets trap moisture and humidity from showers, bathtubs, or sinks that are in close proximity to the cabinet. Heat can also impact medications, and heat is present in bathrooms. Prescription bottles by regulation must meet minimum standards for light (that is why they are amber colored—to prevent damage to the contents by light) and moisture penetration, but can still be susceptible to high-humidity situations.

Storage of medicines in the bathroom is a double-edged sword due to the fact that humidity and heat are present, but it is also a good place to start a routine of taking your medications at a specific time daily. I recommend that if medications are stored in a bathroom, they be placed in a drawer or cupboard away from the sink.

You might also consider storing the medications in the kitchen area, away from heat and moisture. Another option may be to store the medications in bureau drawers in your bedroom or another convenient place for you to remember to take your medications.

## OINTMENTS AND CREAMS

Creams and ointments are very common and useful for many conditions. Your physician may prescribe a cream or ointment for a rash, for insect bites or stings, for eczema or psoriasis, for skin infections, or for types of skin cancer. The type of medications applied to the skin take advantage of the fact that many drugs can penetrate the various layers of the skin and provide relief for many dermatological conditions. Creams, ointments, and gels are termed topical products. They are topical in the sense that they are meant to provide drug therapy for the skin, and not to be absorbed into the blood stream. When considering ointments and creams, several important issues come into play.

A cream is a topical preparation that is water soluble. It is meant to be rubbed into the skin, and it may not be noticeable after it is applied. This is a useful vehicle (method of application) for drugs that need to be rubbed into the skin in order to have an effect.

An ointment is a preparation that is meant to stay on the outer part of the skin; it is greasy by design and is not water soluble unless exposed to soap and water and rinsing. If you have an open sore or other painful condition, the ointment supplies the drug and also can help to protect the skin from further injury. It is an occlusive barrier—it does not allow substances other than the active drug to penetrate the skin. Usually, the ointment is meant to serve as a barrier, to prevent the preparation from washing or rubbing off right away. Ointments may also be applied to orifices of the body and stay in place for a longer period of time. For example, a rectal ointment has the potential to stay in place longer than a cream applied to the rectum.

Some products are also available as a gel formulation. Gels are more than likely alcohol based and can serve as a delivery form for various medications. Gels are clear preparations and are water soluble after washing and rinsing the skin. They may provide an advantage for the application of certain medications that might otherwise be insoluble if delivered via a cream or an ointment.

If your cream or ointment is prescribed to be applied sparingly, what does this mean? Some products such as steroidal anti-inflammatory medications are potent and should be applied lightly. They do not need to be applied in great quantities in order to be effective. If you apply more than a small amount of the product, you will not be provided any additional benefit, and in fact it may be detrimental. They can also be expensive products, and if you apply them in great quantities, you are wasting money and product.

So, how can you tell how much to use? See Figure 10.1 for an example. If it is a steroid cream, this amount can be rubbed over the area. This same admonition holds true if you are applying an antihistamine cream (e.g., diphenhydramine hydrochloride [Benadryl]). You do not need to apply any more than a sparing amount of these products.

If there are multiple areas to cover with either a steroid cream or an antihistamine cream, then you will have to use several of these amounts of the product and spread it around as necessary and instructed by your physician.

If you are applying an antibiotic salve (a salve is just another term for an externally applied cream or ointment), you can apply it more liberally than the sparing amount referred to previously. If you are applying a cream or ointment to a burn area, you will also spread more of the drug than just a small amount.

## TRANSDERMAL PATCHES

Transdermal patches take advantage of the ability of drugs to pass through the skin and into the bloodstream. Various transdermal (across the skin) products are available, and they may include these:

- Clonidine (Catapres-TTS), used for high blood pressure
- Estradiol (Alora, Climara, Esclim), birth control
- Estrogen/progestin (CombiPatch), birth control
- Fentanyl (Duragesic), used for pain relief
- Lidocaine (Lidoderm), used for herpes zoster ("shingles") pain relief
- Nicotine (Nicoderm CQ, Nicotrol, various generic formulations), nicotine replacement therapy for smoking cessation
- Nitroglycerin (Deponit, Minitran, Nitrek, Nitro-Dur), used for angina pectoris
- Oxybutynin (Oxytrol), used for incontinence
- Scopolamine (Transderm Scōp), used for motion sickness
- Testosterone (Testoderm, Androderm), used for androgen insufficiency, hypogonadism

FIGURE 10.1. An example of an "apply sparingly" amount of an ointment or cream.

Specific tips for use, application, and discarding the transdermal patches are important to consider. Each time you apply a new patch, apply it to a different spot than where the patch was last applied. Rotate the site of application so that you do not use the same spot more than once a week. Apply the patch to an area that is clean, hairless, and dry. If the application site has recently been washed with soap, rinse and dry the skin before application. Soap will increase the absorption of some drugs that are contained in transdermal patches (e.g., nicotine is an example of drug which is absorbed more if soap is on the skin at the site of application). Wash your hands after you apply or remove the patch. Remember that the drug can be absorbed through the skin on your fingers as well. Also avoid contact with your eyes, mouth, or other mucous membranes after applying or removing the patches. You can apply the patch to your upper arms, chest, shoulders, hips, or buttocks. Make sure that you are using only one patch at a time. When you apply a new patch, make sure to remove the old patch. Do not leave the patches on for longer than the recommended period; the drugs are designed to be absorbed for a set period of time. Discard the removed patch by folding it onto itself, covering the adhesive area, and placing the folded patch in the pouch in which it came, and then discarding the material away from pets or children. The drugs can be toxic to both children and pets. Patches with adhesive may smell sweet to pets, but the contents can be very harmful to them.

Most of these patches are waterproof, so if you shower or swim, the patches should stay on the skin and remain active. If by chance the patch falls off, you can replace it (on dry skin) by pressing around the circumference of the patch (outer edges). If the patch cannot be retrieved to be applied, then apply a new patch, but remove it at the time the original patch was to be removed and discard it.

Some people experience skin irritation when using any patch. If you are allergic to adhesives or cannot wear other adhesive patches (e.g., adhesive bandages) please let your physician and pharmacist know this. Skin reactions can vary from minor irritation to other more serious skin conditions. Sometimes the irritation can be avoided by simply applying the patch at a different site each time. However, if you notice definite erythema (redness, swollen skin), edema, or papular eruptions (raised nodules or bumps), contact your physician and do not apply any other patches unless instructed to do so. Also, if you notice redness spreading outside the defined area of the patch, contact your physician and pharmacist as well; you may be experiencing an allergic reaction.

## *EYE DROPS*

The membranes of the eye permit drug absorption. Ophthalmic medications include drugs used for glaucoma (increased intraocular pressure), cataracts, conjunctivitis, or other infections (e.g., pink eye).

You should be careful to not touch the tip of the eye dropper, as this can contaminate the contents. The contents are sterile until opened, so you should discard after a period of use. I recommend that products used to treat infections be discarded after the prescribed treatment period defined by your physician. I also suggest that other eye drops be discarded after ninety days or the listed expiration date, whichever comes first.

If you happen to wear contact lenses, do not wear your lenses and apply an eye drop or eye ointment that contains a steroid. This can lead to the steroid perforating your corneas.

Eye ointments are usually applied in the evening. These sterile ophthalmic ointments are specific for use in the eye only. Also, other ointments that are meant for external application should never be applied to the eye. Eye ointments can be difficult to apply. I recommend that you have someone help you with the administration of both eye drops and eye ointments until you can master the technique yourself. For the administration of eye ointments, I suggest that you apply a thin line of the ointment across the inside lower eyelid and try not to touch the eye with the tip of the ointment container. This small ribbon of ointment can then be massaged with your fingers on the outside of your closed eyes.

Drops can be administered in the bottom sac of your eye when you pull the bottom lid out slightly. You can also drop the drops into the corner of your eye toward your nose, then close your eye and gently massage it without rubbing your eye. If you have a puncture wound in the eye, you should not massage the eye. Always ask your eye doctor how the product should be applied. The pharmacist can then help you with the administration techniques when you have the prescription filled at the pharmacy.

## SPECIALTY DOSAGE FORMS

Some drugs are obtained in containers that can make it difficult to view how much medication, if any, is left. Eye drops and nasal sprays are two examples.

The remaining amounts in a metered-dose inhaler (MDI) can also be very difficult to assess. The medication containers (canisters) are not heavy, so the difference between a full, partially full, and empty container may be difficult to figure out. The canisters are metal and light weight, and also are not transparent. So the silver colored canisters are impossible to see through. Instructions for these devices often suggest that you place in water to see if the canister floats (an empty container) or sinks (a more full container). I believe there should be a more accurate method to determine the amount left in these MDIs. I would check to see approximately how many doses are in the container, and count the number of doses that you have used in order to approximate how many doses remain in the container. Ask your pharmacist for other tips on how to tell how much medication is left in your container.

A powder for inhalation for use in asthma to treat airway obstruction and inflammation is packaged in an elaborate dose-delivery container. This drug combination is fluticasone propionate/salmeterol inhalation powder (Advair Diskus). The dosage container is a round container containing a foil pouch with sixty doses contained within the case in blister-wrapped doses. Doses are accessed by holding the container in one hand and placing the thumb of the other hand on the slotted thumb grip. Push your thumb away from you as far as it will go until the mouthpiece appears and snaps into position. At this point, a lever appears that you depress. Depress the lever until it clicks. The powder is now ready to inhale. Do not exhale into the container—it will blow the powder away from you. Every time the lever is pushed back, a dose is ready to be inhaled, and the number counter goes from sixty to zero. This is a very sophisticated delivery device. Patients need to know four things about this device:

1. How to use the container to expose the mouthpiece
2. How to activate the dose with the lever
3. How to inhale the dosage powder
4. How to tell how many doses remain in the container

Even after the full amount of doses is dispensed, the unit will continue to open, the mouthpiece will appear, and the lever can be depressed by clicking it. Thus, the patient can unwittingly think that they are accessing the drug by opening and clicking the lever after the sixty doses have been expended.

The pharmacist should show you where to look for the indicator on the side of the container that lets you know how many doses remain. The container is in a foil pouch that has to be opened. I would recommend that your pharmacist show you how to use the product before you leave the pharmacy.

An unfortunate occurrence has been documented in which a patient continued to use an *empty* Advair Diskus container for five weeks after the counter on the container had reached zero.[1] The patient did not know this and required hospitalization for chronic obstructive pulmonary disease (COPD) symptoms.

This is an example of an exquisitely designed dosage container and dispenser that does not help unless the patient understands how to use it. Here I suggest that if the patient has poor eyesight, he or she should use a magnifying glass to observe how many doses are left by viewing the dose indicator slot on the side of the container. Be sure to obtain a refill of the prescription seven days or so in advance of the depletion of the dispenser to make sure that you have the asthma drug on hand. Also, if someone cannot use his or her hands to open such a container, another person should help with the dose administration.

---

### KEY POINT

*If you cannot use a container or access your medications, ask your pharmacist and physician for alternate containers or drugs that you can access.*

---

These specialized types of dosage containers are examples of well-designed containers that often make it difficult for patients to access therapies. It is one of the biggest reasons why patient compliance is less than what we think it should be. Physicians and pharmacists need to consider the dosage form drugs are dispensed in; if it appears to be too elaborate for a patient to access, other options should be explored that do not appear to be an impediment for patients.

---

**KEY POINT**

*Do not feel that you are the only one who has trouble opening and accessing medication containers. This is a common problem.*

---

## SHARING OR SPLITTING MEDICATIONS

It is not a good idea to share your medications with others. You simply do not have all the information that you need to adequately decide on diagnoses, dosage forms, or whether someone else is allergic to a medication. Also, it is not a good idea to be the recipient of someone else's offer to help you out by sharing medication with you.

---

**KEY POINT**

*It is not a good idea to share your medications with others, or have them share theirs with you.*

---

### Some Pills Should Not Be Split in Half

Certain medications should not be crushed or split. Some products may have a very unpleasant taste unless they are coated, and these are not meant to be split. Other medications may irritate the skin or mucous membranes if split open. Products that are meant to be dissolved over a longer period of time should not be crushed or split. For example, if a tablet is a controlled-release product taken once or twice daily, it should not be crushed or split. The material in the tablet or capsule is coated such that it is slowly released over a period of time. Enteric-coated tablets are meant to be dissolved in the intestines, not in the upper stomach; splitting or crushing them would defeat this purpose.

Some tablets are meant to be dissolved under the tongue. These so-called sublingual tablets (literally translated "under the tongue") also should not be split in half. Other tablets referred to as buccal tablets are meant to dissolve in the side of the mouth and should not be split or cut in any manner.

For the most part, capsules should not be split in half or otherwise opened. Some products are available as capsules that can be opened; your pharmacist will know and be able to provide you with information about specific capsule products that can or cannot be opened. Other capsules, sometimes called liquid-gels, contain liquid medication and should not be split open. The names of these types of dosage forms may be perle (e.g., benzonatate [Tessalon Perles]), gel-cap, soft capsule formulation, or some other name. Always check with your pharmacist if you have questions about whether a capsule can be opened. Your physician may not always know what formulations are available, so your pharmacist is always the best source of information. If your pharmacist has a question, they can always call the physician to clarify the dose and dosage form that you need.

Other medications may not be stable unless in the original dosage form, or they simply cannot be split open. An example of a tablet that cannot be split open is sildenafil citrate (Viagra) 100 mg tablets; it is not possible to split this tablet into two 50 mg tablets without an uneven break of the tablet.

Some tablets have a definite recessed mark on the top of the tablet and can be split in half. This can be done either by using your fingers to split the tablet, or the tablet can be placed on a plate and, using a table knife, gently pried in two. If you are unsure how to do this, ask your pharmacist for assistance or have a family member help you in this task. Use caution when splitting these tablets: do not use excessive force, and make sure your hand or fingers are not under the tablet you are trying to cut in half. You can also purchase a device called a tablet splitter, which eases the process of cutting tablets in half. Ask your pharmacist which device would be best for you.

## OUTDATED DRUGS

Outdated drugs should never be used for any purpose. Drugs are expensive, but this is risky business, and not recommended. Even though the tablet or capsule may appear to be new and show no apparent signs of decay, these drugs must not be used. Drugs for heart ailments, whether they are β-blockers, ACE inhibitors, or nitroglycerin tablets, are examples of drugs with a narrow therapeutic range and any deviance from normal levels obtained with fresh drugs can be life-threatening. The level of the drug in the blood must be within a very narrow range in order for it to be effective.

In other instances, use of outdated drugs may not only have a therapeutic effect but also can be life threatening due to outdated drug breakdown products contained in the dosage form. An example of this occurrence is the use of outdated tetracycline antibiotics. Outdated tetracyclines should never be administered. The breakdown products of outdated tetracycline products are highly toxic to the kidneys (nephrotoxic) and have on occasion produced a kidney disease termed Fanconi-like syndrome.

## OFF-LABEL USES OF DRUGS

In the United States, drugs are required to be carefully used within certain prescribing guidelines. These guidelines stipulate through the FDA-mandated "package insert" what can be written about the drug in the material provided to physicians and pharmacists. The materials that pharmaceutical companies provide to the medical community about their products are strictly controlled.

However, physicians in the United States can write drug prescriptions for indications that are not listed in the approved package insert. These types of prescriptions are termed "off-label" uses of drugs.[2] It is common in the United States for prescriptions to be written in this fashion. In some cases, physicians do not know about these other uses of the drugs from information provided by the drug company, but have read about these uses in medical journal articles.

Not all off-label drugs use is appropriately described. Recently Warner-Lambert was ordered to pay $430 million in fines and civil damages for illegal and fraudulent promotion of unapproved uses of gabapentin (Neurontin).[3] Illegal presentations by company representatives, "conferences" where information was provided, and other avenues were used by Warner-Lambert to illegally promote the drug's off-label uses.[4] Warner-Lambert had promoted gabapentin even when studies had shown it not to be effective in inappropriately claimed indications.[5]

## HOW TO DISPOSE OF UNNECESSARY MEDICATIONS

You will from time to time accumulate extra doses of prescription drugs, bottles with one or two tablets or capsules in them, ointment or cream tubes with small amounts left in them, and so on. The leftover medications may be outdated or simply extra doses that were not taken. The normal inclination is to save these medications for potential future use. I do not suggest doing this; some medications such as antibiotics should be discarded after use and the correct period of dosing in the therapy. It can be confusing to try to manage control of the many small amounts that are left over. Most prescriptions when filled require that the expiration date for the medication be listed on the prescription label. Make sure your pharmacist tells you where to look for this date.

I suggest that you either take the drugs back to your pharmacist for disposal or flush them down the toilet. I do not suggest that you simply dump them in with your normal garbage. It is too easily accessible to pets.

Creams and ointments also are required to have expiration dating; the expiration date for creams and ointments can be found impressed on the bottom "crimp" of the ointment or cream tube. It may be difficult to read, but with a magnifying glass you can spot the date. Here again, if you cannot see where it is, ask you pharmacist to guide you to the spot. I do not worry about using external ointment and cream medications at a point after their initial use and before their expiration dates. They should never be used past the expiration date that is on the actual tube itself, but if the salve is for an infection, and the infection might reoccur at a point in the future, I see nothing wrong with saving the product and using the external cream or ointment in the future. Eye drops are an exception to this. I would not use the eye drops past ninety days of initially opening the container. The sterility of the contents of the product meant for instilling in the eye simply cannot be guaranteed after the product is opened. I would not save them for future use.

In summary, know your drugs, know how they should be stored, and know how to use the containers in which they come. If uses, applications, and access are not clear, always demand answers from your physicians and pharmacists.

# Chapter 11

# How to Help an Aging Parent with Medications

## THE ELDERLY AND NONCOMPLIANCE

The elderly are a class of patients especially affected by noncompliance. Many of you reading this have parents who are seniors, or you are approaching this magic age yourself. The health care system can be difficult for any of us to navigate through; this is doubly so for the elderly.

Compliance in elderly populations is a complex issue.[1] In a qualitative analysis of elderly drug taking, Thompson suggests numerous opportunities to promote the quality use of medicine with seniors, including

- accurate and specific labeling of prescription medications,
- providing adequate drug information, and
- monitoring for adverse affects.[2]

We can fall into a trap when examining the elderly: the trap of stereotyping. Viewing the elderly or seniors as being frail, misusers of medication, and incapable of self-monitoring or self-medicating with accuracy is incorrect. One fact is clear, the elderly are no more noncompliant than other age groups because of their age.[3]

However, many attributes predispose the elderly to noncompliance, including

- social isolation
- chronic diseases
- multiple drug regimens
- complex drug regimens
- severity of disease

Each of these factors would affect anyone adversely. Because the elderly have the potential to have one or more of these risk factors, their ability to be optimally compliant may be compromised.

The results of elderly noncompliance are devastating. Researchers have found that 35 percent of elderly patients are readmitted to hospitals with drug-related problems within six months of initial discharge from a hospital.[4] Drug-related factors were a major reason, rather than a contributing reason, for 50 percent of the readmissions. Not all of these drug-related problems are noncompliance problems, but chances are good that most have a noncompliance component.

Any of the ways to improve compliance listed in Chapter 7 have applicability to the elderly patient. In fact, the elderly may benefit from several of these suggestions to improve compliance. Because of the complexity of the regimens that patients are prescribed, the elderly need special attention.[5] You can provide the help they need to help themselves to be more compliant.

Calling, e-mailing, or visiting senior friends or relatives to remind them to be compliant might take extra time, but it might be just what is needed to help someone comply. If this becomes a routine contact for the individuals, they may be helped a great deal along the path to better compliance.

## *DRUGS THE ELDERLY SHOULD NOT TAKE*

Overmedication of seniors continues to be a problem economically and therapeutically, and it certainly affects individual ability to be compliant.[6] These problems of overmedication apply not only to prescription but also OTC medications.[7] I want to concentrate here on a series of drugs that the elderly should not take without a very good reason. A series of expert panels have been convened to examine drugs that are deemed to be inappropriate for use in the elderly. The most recent panel produced an update in 2003.[8] A physician, Mark Beers, started this process in 1991 with a published paper examining this issue from the perspective of patients in long-term-care facilities.[9] The latest report in 2003 covers seniors in any environment. The disease states examined included the following:

- Heart failure
- Hypertension

- Gastric or duodenal ulcers
- Seizures or epilepsy
- Blood clotting disorders, or those on anticoagulant therapy
- Bladder outflow disorders
- Stress incontinence
- Arrhythmias
- Insomnia
- Parkinson's disease
- Cognitive impairment
- Depression
- Anorexia and malnutrition
- Syncope (fainting or falls)
- Hyponatremia (syndrome of inappropriate antidiuretic hormone [SIADH])
- Seizure disorder
- Obesity
- Chronic obstructive pulmonary disease (COPD)
- Chronic constipation

This list is adapted from a table in the latest revision of the Beers criteria.[10] Drugs were then examined which played a role in either causing the disease or symptom or played a major role in making these conditions worse by their activity. The impact of the offending drugs was then rated as being high or low in severity.[11] Please see Table 11.1 for a corresponding listing of these disease or therapy situations, the drugs that may be inappropriate to use, result, and severity rating that corresponds with these conditions.

I want to stress here that these drugs and diseases are a guide for you to begin discussions with your senior of interest (family, friend, etc.) and his or her physician and pharmacist. These discussions need to revolve around these questions:

- Why is the drug being used?
- Is it absolutely necessary?
- Are there alternatives that make better therapeutic sense?
- Can other drugs be started in place of the offending drugs listed in Table 11.1?

TABLE 11.1. A compilation of potentially inappropriate drugs for use in the elderly and the negative impact they may have on diseases and symptoms.

| Disease or condition affected | Drug(s) to be concerned about | The concern | Severity rating |
|---|---|---|---|
| Heart failure | Disopyramide (Norpace) | Potential to promote fluid retention and exacerbation of heart failure | High |
| Hypertension | Pseudoephedrine (Sudafed), diet pills, and amphetamines | May produce elevation of blood pressure | High |
| Gastric or duodenal ulcers | NSAIDs and aspirin (>325 mg) | May exacerbate existing ulcers or produce new/additional ulcers | High |
| Seizures or epilepsy | Clozapine (Clozaril), chlorpromazine (Thorazine), thioridazine (Mellaril), thiothixene (Navane), and buproprion (Wellbutrin, Zyban) | May lower seizure thresholds | High |
| Blood-clotting disorders or receiving anticoagulant therapy | Aspirin, NSAIDs, dipyridamole (Persantin), ticlopidine (Ticlid), and clopidogrel (Plavix) | May prolong clotting time and elevate INR (international normalized ratio)* values or inhibit platelet aggregation, resulting in an increased potential for bleeding | High |
| Bladder outflow obstruction | Anticholinergics and antihistamines, gastrointestinal antispasmodics, muscle relaxants, oxybutynin (Ditropan), flavoxate (Urispas), anticholinergics, antidepressants, decongestants, and tolterodine (Detrol) | May decrease urinary flow, leading to urinary retention | High |

148

| Condition | Drug(s) | Concern | Rating |
|---|---|---|---|
| Stress incontinence | α-Blockers (doxazosin, prazosin, and terazosin), anticholinergics; tricyclic antidepressants (imipramine hydrochloride, doxepin hydrochloride, and amitriptyline hydrochloride), and long-acting benzodiazepines | May produce polyuria and worsening of incontinence | High |
| Arrhythmias | Tricyclic antidepressants (imipramine hydrochloride, doxepin hydrochloride, and amitriptyline hydrochloride) | Concern due to proarrhythmic effects and ability to produce QT interval changes | High |
| Insomnia | Decongestants (pseudoephedrine), theophylline (Theodur), methylphenidate (Ritalin), MAOIs, and amphetamines | Concern due to CNS stimulant effects | High |
| Parkinson's disease | Metoclopramide (Reglan), conventional antipsychotics, and tacrine (Cognex) | Concern due to their antidopaminergic/cholinergic effects | High |
| Cognitive impairment | Barbiturates, anticholinergics, antispasmodics, and muscle relaxants; CNS stimulants: dextroamphetamine and amphetamine (Adderall), methylphenidate (Ritalin), methamphetamine (Desoxyn), and pemolin | Concern due to CNS-altering effects | High |
| Depression | Long-term benzodiazepine use; sympatholytic agents: methyldopate (Aldomet), reserpine, and guanethidine (Ismelin) | May produce or exacerbate depression | High |
| Anorexia and malnutrition | CNS stimulants: dextroamphetamine and amphetamine (Adderall), methylphenidate (Ritalin), methamphetamine (Desoxyn), pemolin, and fluoxetine (Prozac) | Concern due to appetite-suppressing effects | High |

TABLE 11.1 (continued)

| Disease or condition affected | Drug(s) to be concerned about | The concern | Severity rating |
|---|---|---|---|
| Syncope or falls | Short- to intermediate-acting benzodiazepine and tricyclic antidepressants (imipramine hydrochloride, doxepin hydrochloride, and amitriptyline hydrochloride) | May produce ataxis, impaired psychomotor function, syncope, and additional falls | High |
| SIADH/hyponatremia | SSRIs: fluoxetine (Prozac), citalopram (Celexa), fluvoxamine (Luvox), paroxetine (Paxil), and sertraline (Zoloft) | May exacerbate or cause SIADH | Low |
| Obesity | Olanzapine (Zyprexa) | May stimulate appetite and increase weight gain | Low |
| COPD | Long-acting benzodiazepines: chlordiazepoxide (Librium), chlordiazepoxide and amitriptyline (Limbitrol), clidinium bromide and chlordiazepoxide (Librax), diazepam (Valium), quazepam (Doral), halazepam (Paxipam), and clorazepate (Tranxene); β-blockers: propranolol | CNS adverse effects; may induce respiratory depression; may exacerbate or cause respiratory depression | High |
| Chronic constipation | Calcium channel blockers, anticholinergics, and tricyclic antidepressants (imipramine hydrochloride, doxepin hydrochloride, and amitriptyline hydrochloride) | May exacerbate constipation | Low |

Source: Adapted from Fick DM, Cooper JW, Wade WE, Waller JL, MacLean JR, and Beers MH. Updating the Beers criteria for potentially inappropriate medication use in older adults. Archives of Internal Medicine 2003; 163:2716-2724.

*INR is a conversion unit that takes into account the different sensitivities of thromboplastins and thus provides a standardized value to observe and measure.

You should expect clear answers to these questions. If the answers receive are not clear, please keep the issue open until it can be resolved to your satisfaction. There may be legitimate reasons for some of these drugs to be taken by a senior, and these can be explained to you by the physician. This listing is a guide to use to examine the drugs taken and see if alternatives can be substituted.

Overmedication of seniors continues to be a problem economically, therapeutically, and certainly affects each individual's ability to be compliant. For any patient, and especially for seniors, the fewer drugs that can be taken the better off the person will be. Less is better, and the more that you can do to help the better the outcome will be for the individual(s) involved. Our health care system can be complex to navigate through, and especially so for seniors; lend a hand if you can. Commit yourself to stay involved and help the individual as much as you possibly can.

# Chapter 12

# Summary and Conclusions

## *DOUBLE CHECKING*

If you pick up a prescription at your pharmacy, double check to make sure that you are the one for whom the prescription is written. If the pharmacist asks you what you visited the doctor for, it may mean that it is hard for the pharmacist to decipher the written prescription. It may also mean that they are checking your knowledge about your condition and the medications prescribed for it. Many prescription errors are due to illegible handwriting and lack of follow up by the pharmacist.

## *DOSING*

Be sure you know exactly how to take your medication.[1] In the case of helping another to comply, you both should know what the dose and route of administration are. Always double check that you are taking exactly the dose that you should be.

One of the vexing problems with taking an oral liquid is measuring the dosage accurately. Physicians will write for a dose such as a teaspoonful or five milliliters (5 mL). Household teaspoons are not standardized to hold exactly the same volume of liquid as another teaspoon from another manufacturer. The same holds true for a tablespoon. A tablespoonful is a 15 mL dose, but here again the volume contained in tablespoons varies from manufacturer to manufacturer. My suggested solution is to purchase a liquid measuring cup from your local pharmacy. They all stock these, and it is a good, safe measure for you.

Sometimes a measuring cup will come with a prescription from the pharmacy. These are supplied by the manufacturer and are meant to be used with the medication they come with. Oral dosing syringes are available, too. These syringes allow you to measure the correct dose. Be sure to rinse these oral dosing aids after use and before the next dose administration.

---

**KEY POINT**

*Never use a measuring cup to measure medication that comes in drop form. This could lead to a very large overdose with toxic effects.*

---

Be very cautious about using medications that come with a dropper. These dosage units allow a dose to be provided for you in drops. These droppers *are not* interchangeable from one medication to another. Be especially cautious of *never* using a measuring cup to measure and administer drops to yourself or a loved one.

This admonition holds true for OTC medications as well. One specific problem can occur with acetaminophen (Tylenol) concentrated drops being measured with a dosage cup. The drops are a much more concentrated dose as opposed to acetaminophen (Tylenol) suspension. Never interchange measuring cups with measuring droppers.

## *YOUR PHYSICIAN AND YOU*

The relationship you have with your physician(s) and other caregivers relates to tangible outcomes of care.[2] As was previously noted, the more satisfied that you are with your care, the better the results of that care will be for you. Use your impressions of your caregivers to guide you to stay with them or perhaps consider changing to other providers. You deserve to have clear, jargon-free information provided to you by your caregivers.

## *SKIPPING DOSES TO SAVE MONEY*

Prescriptions are expensive and becoming more so each year. Do what you can to obtain help paying for your medications before you skip doses in order to save money. Do not feel bad if you cannot afford your medications; you are not alone. A recent study found that two-thirds of seniors do not let their physicians or nurses know that they cannot afford their medications.[3] In defense of patients, most physicians do not know how much medications cost and thus are buffered from the burdens their patients experience trying to afford them. It has been shown that there is a 10 percent difference in health status between those that comply and those that try to cut costs by cutting drug dosing.[4] Foregoing compliance with medications, as previously noted, can lead to more expenditures for more drugs, physician visits, emergency room visits, and/or hospitalization.

## MEDICATION ASSISTANCE PROGRAMS

Check with your physician to see if he or she knows of assistance programs that manufacturers sponsor to ease the burden of medication expenses.

### Pharmaceutical Manufacturer Programs

Some manufacturers provide assistance for seniors with low incomes and little or no insurance coverage who take certain medications that they manufacture.[5] The following is a list of some these companies:

- Eli Lilly and Company (http://www.lillyanswers.com/families)
- GlaxoSmithKline (http://bridgestoaccess.gsk.com)
- Novartis (http://www.careplan.novartis.com)
- Pfizer (http://www.pfizerhelpfulanswers.com)
- Together Rx Access (http://www.togetherrxaccess.com)
  - Abbott*
  - AstraZeneca*
  - Aventis*
  - Bristol-Myers Squibb*
  - GlaxoSmithKline*
  - Janssen*
  - LifeScan
  - Novartis*
  - Ortho-McNeill*

*Participants in the Together Rx Program.

- Pfizer
- Takeda
- TAP Pharmaceutical Products

### *State Medication Assistance Programs*

According to the listing on the *AARP Bulletin Online,* the following states have medication assistance programs for seniors with low incomes and no insurance or limited insurance coverage for drugs:

| | |
|---|---|
| Alabama | New Hampshire |
| Arizona | New Jersey |
| California | New Mexico |
| Connecticut | New York |
| Delaware | North Carolina |
| Florida | Ohio |
| Illinois | Oregon |
| Indiana | Pennsylvania |
| Kansas | Rhode Island |
| Maine | South Carolina |
| Maryland | Vermont |
| Michigan | West Virginia |
| Minnesota | Wisconsin |
| Missouri | Wyoming[6] |
| Nevada | |

In addition, the Partnership for Prescription Assistance provides a Web site listing all medication assistance programs (public and private) for patients regardless of age.[7]

## *HELP FOR THE NONCOMPLIANT*

Anything that is offered to help you comply with your medications needs to be tailored to your specific needs.[8] Broad-based programs aimed at everyone may not help you with your medication-taking needs.[9] Make sure your pharmacists and physicians know of your efforts to comply, and ask them to help you with compliance-enhancing suggestions. The more you are an active participant in the medication-taking process the better the chances for your success.[10] Providing help to you may be labor intensive and cost more, but the savings derived make it worthwhile.

## Concluding Comment for Us All

You may be helped by some of the things mentioned in this text. However, if you have tried one or more of these suggestions and still have trouble complying, keep trying and do not give up. We all can do better with taking our medications. The health of you and others and the health care system depends on better compliance by us all.

# Appendix

# Web Site Resources

## *Health on the Internet*

Before I list the specific Web sites, I want to say a little about Web sites and information that appears on the Internet. Not everything that is on the Internet provides accurate information. Some of what appears is not worth reading and certainly is suspect regarding the accuracy of the materials presented. A foundation called Health on the Net (HON) will help guide you to accurate information. The mission of HON, as listed on their Web site,

> is to guide the growing community of health care consumers and providers on the World Wide Web to sound, reliable medical information and expertise. In this way, HON seeks to contribute to better, more accessible and cost-effective health care.

If the Web site that you are examining has the seal of approval from HON, the site has been evaluated for accuracy. HON provides a code of conduct for Web information. It can be found at <http://www.hon.ch/HONCODE/conduct.html>.

## *Specific Web Sites with Information of Use to Seniors and Families*

- The National Council on Aging
  http://www.ncoa.org
  NCOA is a national voice and powerful advocate for public policies that promote healthy aging.
- Access to Benefits Coalition (Rx access for those who need them most)
  http://www.accesstobenefits.org
  Currently more than seventy national nonprofit members belong to the Access to Benefits Coalition, sharing the interest of helping low-income Medicare beneficiaries find the public and private prescrip-

tion savings programs they need to maintain their health and improve the quality of their lives.
- WebMD Health
  http://my.webmd.com/medical_information/condition_centers/default.htm
  http://my.webmd.com/medical_information/medicare_rx_benefits/default.htm
- The Mayo Clinic
  http://www.mayoclinic.com/index.cfm

## U.S. Government Healthfinder Affiliated Organizations and Web Sites

- http://www.healthfinder.gov/organizations/
- Agency for Healthcare Research and Quality—Five Steps to Safer Health Care
  http://www.healthfinder.gov/

## Several Disease-Based National Organization Web Sites

- American Heart Association
  http://www.americanheart.org
- American Diabetes Association
  http://www.diabetes.org
- American Cancer Society
  http://www.cancer.org
- American Lung Association
  http://www.lungusa.org

## Web Sites for Parents and Children

- American Academy of Pediatrics
  www.aap.org
- Children's Hospital of Wisconsin
  www.chw.org
- KidsGrowth (a site for parents developed by pediatricians)
  www.kidsgrowth.com
- Mayo Clinic
  www.mayoclinic.com
- Medem—Physician Patient Network
  www.medem.com

- U.S. National Institutes of Health, National Library of Medicine, Medline Plus Child Development site
  www.nlm.nih.gov/medlineplus/childdevelopment.html
- Nemours Foundation
  www.kidshealth.org
- University of Iowa Health Care Virtual Hospital site
  www.vh.org
- WebMD
  http://www.webmd.com
  WebMD is a for-profit Internet site with the following statement appearing on the site: "WebMD Health is the leading provider of online information, educational services and communities for physicians and consumers."

## Web Sites for More Information About Drugs

I recommend only those sites that provide unbiased drug information for consumers. Many Web sites provide drug information, but do it for the purposes of encouraging the consumer to purchase medications online.

- National Library of Medicine and National Institutes of Health
  http://www.nlm.nih.gov/medlineplus/druginformation.html
  http://medlineplus.gov/esp/
  (Both Español and English versions)
- The Mayo Clinic
  http://www.mayoclinic.com/index.cfm
- The Herbal Research Foundation
  http://www.herbs.org/
  The Herbal Research Foundation supports a Web site with comprehensive information about herbs and herbal supplements.

## The U.S. Food and Drug Administration Web Sites for Consumer Education and Information

- http://www.fda.gov/cder/consumerinfo/DPAdefault.htm
  The FDA is committed to providing consumers with information on prescription, generic, and over-the-counter drug products. The Center for Drug Evaluation and Research has developed numerous public service campaigns and announcements to help you make informed decisions about using medicines.
- http://www.asyouage.samhsa.gov/Default.aspx
  U.S. FDA Web site on the dangers of mixing drugs and alcohol

- http://www.fda.gov/cder/consumerinfo/dontBuyonNet.htm
  U.S. FDA Web site on several drugs that should not be purchased from non-U.S. sources
- http://vm.cfsan.fda.gov/~dms/supplmnt.html
  U.S. FDA information on nutritional supplements

# Notes

## Chapter 1

1. Withering W. *An account of the foxglove and some of its medicinal uses.* Birmingham, UK: M. Swinney, 1785.

2. Thompson CJS. *The mystery and art of the apothecary.* Philadelphia: Lippincott, 1929.

3. Kremers E, Urdang G, Sonnedecker G. *Kremers and Urdang's history of pharmacy.* Philadelphia: Lippincott, 1963.

4. Thompson, *The mystery and art of the apothecary.*

5. Institute for Safe Medication Practices. Key questions. Available online at <http://www.ismp.org/Consumer/ Brochure.html>.

6. Bullman R. Educate before you medicate: Your lifeline for safe medicine use. *FDA Consumer* 2001; 35(5):40.

7. Ibid.

## Chapter 2

1. Burt CW. National trends in use of medications in office-based practices, 1985-1999. *Health Affairs* 2002; 21(4):206-214.

2. Ekedahl A, Manson N. Unclaimed prescriptions after automated prescription transmittals to pharmacies. *Pharmacy World & Science* 2004; 26:26-31.

3. Johnson JA, Bootman JL. Drug-related morbidity and mortality. A cost of illness model. *Archives of Internal Medicine* 1995; 155(18):1949-1956.

4. Mojtabai R, Olfson M. Medication costs, adherence, and health outcomes among Medicare beneficiaries. *Health Affairs* 2003; 22(4):220-229.

5. Kaufman FR, Funnell M. *American Diabetes Association complete guide to diabetes.* New York: Bantam Dell Publishing, 2003.

6. Paul L, Nagle B (eds.). *Medication guidebook for healthy aging.* Franklin Lakes, NJ: Merck-Medco Managed Care, L.L.C., 2001.

7. Young L. *The book of the heart.* New York: Doubleday, 2003.

8. Fields LE, Burt VL, Cutler JA, Hughes J, Roccella EJ, and Sorlie P. The burden of adult hypertension in the United States 1999 to 2000, a rising tide. *Hypertension* 2004; 44:1-7.

9. Institute for the Future (ed.). Health care providers themes of the future delivery system. In *Health and health care 2010: The forecast, the challenge,* Second edition. San Francisco, CA: Jossey-Bass, 2003, p. 83.

## Chapter 3

1. Elgin SH. *The last word on the gentle art of verbal self-defense.* New York: Prentice-Hall, 1987, p. 125.

2. Hart J. Court upholds prison term for Courtney. *The Kansas City Star,* April 6, 2004; p. B2.

3. Associated Press. More arrested in pharmaceutical black market ring. Real Cities Network. Available online at <http://www.realcities.com/mld/realcities/9620386.htm>.

4. O'Neil J. Hazards in the medicine cabinet. *The New York Times,* Vital signs, August 10, 2004; p. F6.

5. Fick DM, Cooper JW, Wade WE, Waller J, MacLean R, Beers MH. Updating the Beers criteria for potentially inappropriate medication use in older adults. *Archives of Internal Medicine* 2003; 163:2716-2724.

6. Ukens C. Confrontation at the counter. *Drug Topics,* July 26, 2004; 148:26. Available online at <www.drugtopics.com>.

7. Spake A. Fake drugs, real worries: High prices and the Internet are making U.S. patients easy prey. *U.S. News & World Report,* September 20, 2004. Available online at <http://www.usnews.com/usnews/health/articles/040920/20internet.htm>.

## Chapter 4

1. U.S. Food and Drug Administration. Illnesses and injuries associated with the use of selected dietary supplements. In *Unsubstantiated claims and documented health hazards in the dietary supplement marketplace.* Washington, DC: United States Food and Drug Administration, Center for Food Safety and Applied Nutrition, 1993. Available online at <http://www.cfsan.fda.gov/~dms/ds-ill.html>. See update link at bottom of Web page.

2. Ibid.

3. Ibid.

4. Ibid.

5. Ibid.

6. U.S. Food and Drug Administration. FDA warns consumers about counterfeit drugs purchased in Mexico. *FDA Talk Paper* T04-28, July, 2004. Available online at <http://www.fda.gov/bbs/topics/ANSWERS/2004/ANS01303.html>.

7. U.S. Food and Drug Administration. FDA Consumer Alert: Don't buy these drugs over the Internet or from foreign sources. U.S. FDA, Center for Drug Evaluation and Research, 2003, 2004. Available online at <www.fda.gov/cder/consumerinfo/dontBuyonNet.htm>.

## Chapter 5

1. Lacy CF, Armstrong LL, Goldman MP, Lance L. *Lexi-Comp's Drug Information Handbook 2004-2005,* Twelfth Edition. Hudson, OH: Lexi-Comp Inc., 2004, p. 327.

2. Ibid., p. 945.

3. Ibid., p. 1505.

4. Ibid., p. 349.

5. Ibid., p. 1312.

6. Ibid.

7. Ibid., p. 1313.

8. New drug interaction warnings for the antidepressant trazadone (DESYREL). *Worst Pills Best Pills* 2004; 10(8):63.

9. Lacy et al., *Lexi-Comp's Drug Information Handbook,* p. 83.

10. Ibid.

11. Ibid., p. 1342.

12. Ibid., p. 1462.

13. Ibid., p. 724.

14. Ibid.

15. Anonymous. Drug interaction reminder—Fluoroquinolone antibiotics and the anticoagulant (blood thinner) warfarin (Coumadin). *Worst Pills Best Pills* 2004; 10(9):70-71.

16. Ibid.

17. Ibid.

18. Lacy et al., *Lexi-Comp's Drug Information Handbook,* p. 523.

19. Ibid.; Abramowicz M (ed.). Drugs for lipids. *Treatment Guidelines* March 2005; 3(31):15-22.

20. Lacy et al., *Lexi-Comp's Drug Information Handbook,* p. 1026.

21. The Medical Letter. *Medical letter handbook of adverse drug interactions.* New Rochelle, NY: The Medical Letter, 2001; p. 69.

22. Lacy et al., *Lexi-Comp's Drug Information Handbook,* p. 1521.

23. Ibid., p. 202.

24. Ibid., p. 775.

25. Ibid., p. 569.

26. Ibid., p. 1521.

27. Do NSAIDs interfere with the cardioprotective effects of aspirin? *The Medical Letter,* August 2, 2004; 46(1188):61-62; Lewis JD. Debate continues over existence, importance of aspirin-NSAID interaction. *APhA DrugInfoLine* 2004; 5(7):3.

28. Lewis, Debate continues over aspirin-NSAID interaction, p. 3.

29. Ibid.

30. Drug interactions with St. John's wort. *The Medical Letter,* June 26, 2000; 1081:56.

31. Ibid.

32. Ibid.

33. Ibid.

34. Ibid.

35. Ibid.

36. Ibid.

37. Ibid.; Wood AJJ. Herbal remedies. *New England Journal of Medicine* 2002; 347(25):2046-2056.

38. The University of Michigan Health System. Selected herb-drug interactions. Available online at <http://www.med.umich.edu/1libr/aha/umherb01.htm>.

39. Ibid.

40. Ibid.

41. Ibid.

42. Lambrecht JE, Hamilton W, Rabinovich A. A review of herb-drug interactions: Documented and theoretical. *U.S. Pharmacist* 2000; 25(8):42, 44-46, 48-50, 53.

43. The University of Michigan Health System, Selected herb-drug interactions.

44. Ibid.

45. Ibid.

46. Ibid.

47. Lambrecht, Hamilton, and Rabinovich, A review of herb-drug interactions.

48. Wood, Herbal remedies.

49. The University of Michigan Health System, Selected herb-drug interactions.

50. Lambrecht, Hamilton, and Rabinovich, A review of herb-drug interactions.

51. Ibid.

52. Lacy et al., *Lexi-Comp's Drug Information Handbook,* p. 1462.

53. Almeida JC, Grimsley EW. Coma from the health food store: Interaction between kava kava and alprazolam. *Annals of Internal Medicine* 1996; 125:940-941.

54. Wood, Herbal remedies.

55. The University of Michigan Health System, Selected herb-drug interactions.

56. Lacy et al., *Lexi-Comp's Drug Information Handbook,* pp. 1342, 1462.

57. The University of Michigan Health System, Selected herb-drug interactions.

58. Ibid.

59. Ibid.; Lambrecht et al., A review of herb-drug interactions.

60. The University of Michigan Health System, Selected herb-drug interactions.

61. Miller LG. Herbal medicinals: Selected clinical considerations focusing on known or potential drug-herb interactions. *Archives of Internal Medicine* 1998; 158(20):2200-2211.

62. The University of Michigan Health System, Selected herb-drug interactions.

63. Ibid.

64. Wood, Herbal remedies.

65. *Interactions: The IBIS Guide to Drug-Herb and Drug-Nutrient Interactions,* Version 1998-1999, Integrated Medical Arts Group, Inc. Available online at <http://ibismedical.com/Interactions.html>.

66. Goldman P. Herbal medicines today and the roots of modern pharmacology. *Annals of Internal Medicine* 2001; 135(8):594-600.

67. Fincham JE. Smoking cessation: Treatment options and the pharmacist's role. *American Pharmacy* 1992; NS32 (5):62-71.

68. Lipman A. How smoking interferes with drug therapy. *Modern Medicine* 1985; 53:141-142; Pelkonen O, Maenpaa J, Taavitsainen P, Rautio A, Raunio H. Inhibition and induction of human cytochrome P450 (CYP) enzymes. *Xenobiotica* 1998; 28:1203-1253; Schein JR. Cigarette smoking and clinically significant drug interactions. *Annals of Pharmacotherapy* 1995; 29:1139-1148; Shoaf SE, Linnoila M. Interaction of ethanol and smoking on the pharmacokinetics and pharmacodynamics of psychotropic medications. *Psychopharmacology Bulletin* 1991; 27:577-594.

69. Dahan A, Altman H. Food-drug interaction: Grapefruit juice augments drug bioavailability/mechanism, extent and relevance. *European Journal of Clinical Nutrition* 2004; 58(1):1-9; Shaw LK. Putting drug interactions with grapefruit juice in perspective. *Pharmacy Times* 2003. Available online at <http://www.pharmacy times.com/article.cfm?ID=258>.

70. Dahan and Altman, Food-drug interaction.

71. Shaw, Putting drug interactions in perspective.

72. Dahan and Altman, Food-drug interaction; Shaw, Putting drug interactions in perspective.

73. Ibid.

74. Ibid.

75. Ibid.

76. Ibid.

## *Chapter 6*

1. American Medical Association. Records of physicians: Information and patients. Policy E-7.02. Issued prior to April 1977; Updated June 1994. Available online at <http://www.ama-assn.org/ama/pub/category/8378.html>.

2. Ibid.

3. National Institutes of Health. HIPAA Privacy Rule: Information for researchers. Available online at <http://privacyruleandresearch.nih.gov/pr_07.asp>.

4. Steinhauer J. Justice department finds success chasing health care fraud. *The New York Times,* January 23, 2001; p. A19.

5. Committee on Maintaining Privacy and Security in Health Care Applications of the National Information Infrastructure. *For the record, protecting electronic health information.* Washington, DC: National Academy Press, 1997.

6. Weslander E. Web site helps prevent ID theft. *Lawrence Journal-World,* August 14, 2004. Available online at <http://www.ljworld.com/section/kutoday2004d/story/178089>.

## *Chapter 7*

1. Dunbar JM, Marshall GD, Hovell MF. Behavioral strategies for improving compliance. In RB Haynes, DW Taylor, DL Sacket (eds.). *Compliance in health care.* Baltimore: The Johns Hopkins University Press, 1979, pp. 174-190.

2. Sabaté E (ed.). *Adherence to long-term therapies: Evidence for action.* Geneva, Switzerland: World Health Organization, 2003; Haynes RB, McDonald HP, Garg AX. Helping patients follow prescribed treatment: Clinical applications. *JAMA* 2002; 288(22):2880-2883.

3. McDonald HP, Garg AX, Haynes RB. Interventions to enhance patient adherence to medication prescriptions: Scientific review. *JAMA* 2002; 288(22):2868-2879.

4. Peterson AM, Takiya L, Finley R. Meta-analysis of trials of interventions to improve medication adherence. *American Journal of Health-System Pharmacy* 2003; 60(7):657-665.

5. Fincham JE. The drug-use process. In JE Fincham and AI Wertheimer (eds.). *Pharmacy and the U.S. health care system,* Second edition. Binghamton, NY: The Haworth Press, 1998, pp. 395-438.

6. Fincham JE, Wertheimer AI. Using the health belief model to predict initial drug therapy defaulting. *Social Science and Medicine* 1985; 20(1):101-105.

7. Bultman DC, Svarstad BL. Effects of physician communication style on client medication beliefs and adherence with antidepressant treatment. *Social Science and Medicine* 2000; 40:173-185.

8. Stevenson F, Barry C, Britten N, Barber N, Bradley CP. Doctor-patient communication about drugs: The evidence for shared decision making. *Social Science & Medicine* 2000; 50:829-840.

9. Segarra J, DeStefano JJ, Davis RH. Streamlining outpatient prescription dispensing utilizing prescriber order entry. *ASHP Midyear Clinical Meeting* 1991; 26(Dec):P-425D.

10. Forcinio H. Packaging solutions that help patient compliance. *The Journal of Pharmacy Technology* 1993; 17(Mar):44, 46, 48, 50.

11. Carr-Lopez SM, Mallett MS, Morse T. Tablet splitter: Barrier to compliance or cost-saving instrument? *American Journal of Health-System Pharmacy* 1995; 52(Dec 1):2707-2708.

12. Perri M, Martin BC, Pritchard FL. Improving medication compliance: Practical intervention. *The Journal of Pharmacy Technology* 1995; 11(Jul-Aug):167-172.

13. Urquhart J. When outpatient drug treatment fails: Identifying noncompliers as a cost-containment tool. *Medical Interface* 1993; 6(Apr):65-67, 71-73.

14. Wingender W, Kuppers J. Bayer compliance device. *Drug Information Journal* 1993; 27(4):1103-1106.

15. Tiano FJ. Compliant packaging. *Clinical Research Practices and Regulatory Affairs* 1994; 11(1):39-46.

16. Forcinio H. Packaging solutions that help patient compliance. *The Journal of Pharmacy Technology* 1993; 17(Mar):44, 46, 48, 50.

17. Rigby M. Pharmaceutical packaging can induce confusion. *British Medical Journal* 2002; 324:679.

## *Chapter 8*

1. Bellenir K (ed.). *Diabetes sourcebook: Basic consumer health information about type 1 diabetes (insulin-dependent or juvenile-onset diabetes), type 2 diabetes (noninsulin-dependent or adult)* (Health Reference Series, Second edition). Detroit: Omnigraphics, 1998.

2. Whitaker J. *Reversing hypertension: A vital new program to prevent, treat, and reduce high blood pressure.* New York: Warner Books, 2001.

3. Glickman R. *Optimal thinking: How to be your best self.* Hoboken, NJ: John Wiley & Sons, Inc., 2002, pp. 156-158.

## *Chapter 9*

1. Burt CW. National trends in use of medications in office-based practices, 1985-1999. *Health Affairs* 2002; 21(4):206-214.

## Chapter 10

1. Institute for Safe Medication Practices. Safety briefs: Check the indicator. *ISMP Medication Safety Alert!* 2004; 3(9):1-4.
2. American Academy of Pediatrics, Committee on Drugs. Uses of drugs not described in the package insert (off-label uses). *Pediatrics* 2002; 110(1):181-183.
3. Larkin M. Warner-Lambert found guilty of promoting Neurontin off label. *The Lancet Neurology* 2004; 3(7):387.
4. Anonymous. Drug maker to pay $430 million in fines, civil damages. *FDA Consumer* 2004; July-Aug:36-37.
5. Ibid.

## Chapter 11

1. Herrier RN. Medication compliance in the elderly. *Journal of Pharmacy Practice* 1995; 8(Oct):232-244.
2. Thompson S. Opinions and prescription medication use practices among the non-institutionalised elderly. Doctoral thesis, Victorian College of Pharmacy, Monash University, Melbourne, Victoria, Australia, 1996.
3. Lorence L, Branthwaite A. Are older adults less compliant with prescribed medication than younger adults? *British Journal of Clinical Psychology* 1993; 32: 485-492.
4. Bero LA, Lipton HL, Bird JA. Characterization of geriatric drug-related hospital readmissions. *Medical Care* 1991; 29(Oct):989-1003.
5. Meredith PA. Enhancing patients' compliance. *British Medical Journal* 1998; 316:393-394.
6. Cohen JS. Avoiding adverse reactions. *Geriatrics* 2000; 55(2):54-64.
7. Fincham JE. Over-the-counter drug use and misuse by the ambulatory elderly: A review of the literature. *Journal of Geriatric Drug Therapy* 1986; 1(2):3-22.
8. Fick DM, Cooper JW, Wade WE, Waller JL, MacLean JR, Beers MH. Updating the Beers criteria for potentially inappropriate medication use in older adults. *Archives of Internal Medicine* 2003; 163:2716-2724.
9. Beers MH, Ouslander JG, Rollingher J, Reuben DB, Beck JC. Explicit criteria for determining inappropriate medication use in nursing home residents. *Archives of Internal Medicine* 1991; 151:1825-1832.
10. Fick et al., Updating the Beers criteria.
11. Ibid.

## Chapter 12

1. See Institute for Safe Medication Practices: Be an informed consumer, Key questions, and What you can do. Available online at <http://www.ismp.org/Consumer/Brochure.html>.
2. Kim SS, Kaplowitz S, Johnston MV. The effects of physician empathy on patient satisfaction and compliance. *Evaluation & the Health Professions* 2004; 27(3):237-251.

3. Piette JD, Heisler M, Wagner TH. Cost-related medication underuse: Do patients with chronic illnesses tell their doctors? *Archives of Internal Medicine* 2004; 164:1749-1755.

4. Heisler M, Langa K, Eby EL, Fendrick AM, Kabeto MU, Piette JD. The health effects of restricting prescription medication use because of cost. *Medical Care* 2004; 42(7):626-634.

5. Together Rx Access. Savings for qualified individuals and families without prescription coverage. 2005. Available online at <http://www.togetherrxaccess.com>.

6. See Gearon CJ. State-by-state, plan-by-plan list of pharmacy assistance programs. *AARP Bulletin* Online, 2004. Available online at <http://www.aarp.org/bulletin/yourmoney/Articles/statebystate.html>.

7. Partnership for Prescription Assistance. Welcome to PPARx.org. 2005. Available online at <https://www.pparx.org/Intro.php>.

8. Meredith PA. Enhancing patients' compliance. *British Medical Journal* 1998; 316:393-394.

9. Partnership for Prescription Assistance. Welcome to PPARx.org. 2005. Available online at <https://www.pparx.org/Intro.php>.

10. Stevenson FA, Barry CA, Britten N, Barber N, Bradley CP. Doctor-patient communication about drugs: The evidence for shared decision making. *Social Science & Medicine* 2000; 50:829-840.

# Index

Page numbers followed by the letter "t" indicate tables; those followed by the letter "f" indicate figures; and those followed by the letter "e" indicate exhibits.

## Order a copy of this book with this form or online at:
http://www.haworthpress.com/store/product.asp?sku=5579

# TAKING YOUR MEDICINE
# A Guide to Medication Regimens and Compliance
# for Patients and Caregivers

_____in hardbound at $39.95 (ISBN-13: 978-0-7890-2858-7; ISBN-10: 0-7890-2858-1)

_____in softbound at $22.95 (ISBN-13: 978-0-7890-2859-4; ISBN-10: 0-7890-2859-X)

Or order online and use special offer code HEC25 in the shopping cart.

COST OF BOOKS_____

POSTAGE & HANDLING_____
(US: $4.00 for first book & $1.50
for each additional book)
(Outside US: $5.00 for first book
& $2.00 for each additional book)

SUBTOTAL_____

IN CANADA: ADD 7% GST_____

STATE TAX_____
(NJ, NY, OH, MN, CA, IL, IN, PA, & SD
residents, add appropriate local sales tax)

FINAL TOTAL_____
(If paying in Canadian funds,
convert using the current
exchange rate, UNESCO
coupons welcome)

☐ **BILL ME LATER:** (Bill-me option is good on
US/Canada/Mexico orders only; not good to
jobbers, wholesalers, or subscription agencies.)
☐ Check here if billing address is different from
shipping address and attach purchase order and
billing address information.

Signature_____

☐ **PAYMENT ENCLOSED: $_____**

☐ **PLEASE CHARGE TO MY CREDIT CARD.**

☐ Visa ☐ MasterCard ☐ AmEx ☐ Discover
☐ Diner's Club ☐ Eurocard ☐ JCB

Account # _____

Exp. Date_____

Signature_____

Prices in US dollars and subject to change without notice.

NAME_____

INSTITUTION_____

ADDRESS_____

CITY_____

STATE/ZIP_____

COUNTRY_____ COUNTY (NY residents only)_____

TEL_____ FAX_____

E-MAIL_____

May we use your e-mail address for confirmations and other types of information? ☐ Yes ☐ No
We appreciate receiving your e-mail address and fax number. Haworth would like to e-mail or fax special
discount offers to you, as a preferred customer. **We will never share, rent, or exchange your e-mail address
or fax number.** We regard such actions as an invasion of your privacy.

*Order From Your Local Bookstore or Directly From*
**The Haworth Press, Inc.**
10 Alice Street, Binghamton, New York 13904-1580 • USA
TELEPHONE: 1-800-HAWORTH (1-800-429-6784) / Outside US/Canada: (607) 722-5857
FAX: 1-800-895-0582 / Outside US/Canada: (607) 771-0012
E-mail to: orders@haworthpress.com

**For orders outside US and Canada,** you may wish to order through your local
sales representative, distributor, or bookseller.
For information, see http://haworthpress.com/distributors

*(Discounts are available for individual orders in US and Canada only, not booksellers/distributors.)*

PLEASE PHOTOCOPY THIS FORM FOR YOUR PERSONAL USE.
http://www.HaworthPress.com                                    BOF04